The Children of Africa Confront AIDS

This series of publications on Africa, Latin America, Southeast Asia, and Global and Comparative Studies is designed to present significant research, translation, and opinion to area specialists and to a wide community of persons interested in world affairs. The editor seeks manuscripts of quality on any subject and can usually make a decision regarding publication within three months of receipt of the original work. Production methods generally permit a work to appear within one year of acceptance. The editor works closely with authors to produce a high-quality book. The series appears in a paperback format and is distributed worldwide. For more information, contact the executive editor at Ohio University Press, Scott Quadrangle, University Terrace, Athens, Ohio 45701.

Executive editor: Gillian Berchowitz
AREA CONSULTANTS
Africa: Diane M. Ciekawy
Latin America: Thomas Walker
Southeast Asia: William H. Frederick
Global and Comparative Studies: Ann R. Tickamyer

The Ohio University Research in International Studies series is published for the Center for International Studies by Ohio University Press. The views expressed in individual volumes are those of the authors and should not be considered to represent the policies or beliefs of the Center for International Studies, Ohio University Press, or Ohio University.

The Children of Africa Confront AIDS

From Vulnerability to Possibility

Edited by

Arvind Singhal

and

W. Stephen Howard

Ohio University Research in International Studies
Africa Series No. 80
Ohio University Press
Athens

© 2003 by the Center for International Studies
Ohio University
Printed in the United States of America
All rights reserved

12 11 10 09 08 07 06 05 04 03   5 4 3 2 1

The books in the Ohio University Research in International Studies Series
are printed on acid-free paper ∞

Published in the United States of America by Ohio University Press,
Athens, Ohio 45701

Library of Congress Cataloging-in-Publication Data

The children of Africa confront AIDS : from vulnerability to possibility / edited by Arvind Singhal and W. Stephen Howard.
    p. cm. – (Ohio University research in international studies. Africa series ; no. 80)
    Includes bibliographical references and index.
    ISBN 0-89680-232-9 (pbk. : alk. paper)
    1. AIDS (Disease) in children—Africa.   2. Children of AIDS patients—Africa.
3. Orphans—Africa.   I. Singhal, Arvind, 1962– II. Howard, W. Stephen.
III. Research in international studies. Africa series ; no. 80.

RJ387.A25C485 2003
618.92'9792'0096—dc21   2003056311

Contents

Section 2: Coping

Section 3: Courage

Section 4: Possibility

Illustrations

Foreword

The statistics overwhelm the language and confound the imagination. Humankind has never known a tragedy of these proportions. Sub-Saharan Africa, where 83 percent of all AIDS deaths and 71 percent of HIV infections occur, has been described as Ground Zero. But terms like New Holocaust and Ground Zero belong to another world, whatever the images of suffering connected to them. They belong to the world of the powerful, and in our desperation to have our tragedy of unspeakable proportions recognized we invoke words that we hope will resonate with the powerful. It's as if our own pain can only be legitimized in the shadow of theirs.

Stephen Lewis of UNAIDS recently demanded that "those who watch [this pandemic] unfold with a kind of pathological equanimity must be held to account" and suggested that "there may yet come a day when we have peacetime tribunals to deal with this particular version of crimes against humanity." On the morning of September 11, one of the local Starbucks in the vicinity of Ground Zero actually sold water to distraught people fleeing the disaster. The sales lasted for only a short while and then the sickness of it all sank in and the company apologized. Will a time come when companies will be held accountable for having profiteered on the blood of people because they insisted on putting profits and patents before people and patients? When will the sickness of it all sink in?

Like no other pandemic, HIV/AIDS reflects the games of the powerful on the one hand and the survival mechanisms and cries of the powerless on the other. Some African governments refuse to do the doable, invoking unconvincing arguments about budgetary constraints—unconvincing because their defense budgets are there for all to see. Rather than engaging in frontal assault on reckless sexual behavior that not infrequently involves violence and rape, we find it more convenient to seek refuge in conspiracy theories. White society ascribes the crisis to "black promiscuity"; blacks, to white pharmaceutical companies; straight people, to "homosexual promiscuity"; religious people, to those with "loose morals"; the North, to the "decadence" of the South.

HIV/AIDS is the ultimate in othering. Alas there is no North or South, and I have yet to come across a "real" black person or white person. Sometimes when I wash the body of someone who has died of AIDS I weep and ask myself why—particularly when I did not know the deceased. I cry for myself, my own selfhood, which comprises so many others; I am the other, for otherness is a condition of selfhood; I am who I am because of you.

This is not the time for homily or one-upmanship (and for once, gender-biased language works just fine with me). When I arrive at the scene of an accident and I witness the injured struggling for their lives, what does it say about me when I rush to smell their breath for alcohol, walk off into the desert of indifference, and use the opportunity to crow about my being a teetotaler? Surely my humanity dies along with those victims.

If Not for Yourself, then at Least for the Children

While no adult who is HIV-positive has asked for it, they are not as innocent as the children—the utterly voiceless, the unspeakably vulnerable. The children have only me and you to depend on. In each of these children we have a reflection of where we were once upon a time and, but for the grace of God, it could have been me yesterday or my children tomorrow.

This volume deals with the children of Africa—how their lives and deaths are affecting development and democracy in that continent as well as their vulnerability in the face of war and poverty and the often related sexual violence. These chapters are not tales of lamentation but of hope and courage; From Zimbabwe to Ghana, from Kenya to South Africa, come stories and strategies for reducing vulnerability and sustaining survival and solidarity.

There is life after HIV. For years now, in the more developed countries and among affluent individuals in poorer countries, it is common for HIV-positive persons to be living with the virus for twenty years or more. Why should it be any different for the children of Africa? In the years of our struggle against apartheid in South Africa, our slogan was Mobilize or Starve! Sadly this becomes our call again—for HIV-positive people to mobilize or perish; and as in that struggle, where we slew the beast of apartheid along with white comrades who realized that that their humanity was being tested by their involvement with us or their refusal to get involved, so too will we overcome when people who are not infected realize that all of us are affected.

—FARID ESACK

Preface and Acknowledgments

Kami is a five-year-old, mustard-colored, bearlike puppet (very similar to a Muppet) sporting a mop of brown hair and a beaded blue vest. She loves nature, telling stories, and playing with children. Kami's parents died when she was young and she is HIV-positive.

On September 30, 2002, the furry Kami joined the cast of *Takalani Sesame,* South Africa's version of *Sesame Street,* to help three- to seven-year-olds (and their families) understand and cope with HIV and AIDS. Takalani means "be happy" in the local Venda language, and Kami's name is derived from the Tswana word for acceptance. In a world where HIV-positive children are often isolated, demonized, and victimized, Kami symbolizes hope, possibility, and understanding. She embodies African children's vulnerability to HIV and AIDS,[1] including the possibilities of compassionately confronting the pandemic. This book is about the Kamis of Africa, the continent hardest hit by the HIV/AIDS pandemic.

This volume, the first book produced by the Institute for the African Child (IAC), was inspired by our 2002 conference "HIV/AIDS and the African Child: Health Challenges, Educational Possibilities." Founded in 1998 at Ohio University, the IAC is a group of social scientists, communication specialists, and educational and medical scientists working together, across disciplines and issues, to focus on the world's most marginalized of population groups, the children of Africa.

Our perspectives here are those of a sociologist (Howard) and a communication scholar (Singhal) who are trying to understand the context of the AIDS plague and its impact on changing African societies and institutions, and on Africa's future, Africa's children. We are seeing in the AIDS crisis manifestations of leadership for positive social change, and an increasingly committed leadership that has children as its motivation and, in some dramatic cases, its fulcrum.

In this book we are trying to participate in conversations between humanitarian and political activism and academic debates, asking, What shall we do? in African contexts ranging from the classroom in Botswana to youth groups in Kenya and Ghana. Our authors describe HIV/AIDS in its macro contexts: the continent's democratization movements and the vulnerability of children caught in civil conflicts. On a micro scale we see children not only as victims of rural poverty, but as beneficiaries of youth organizations and other agencies working on the ground. Media campaigns have also become highly visible interventions and detailed examples are provided here. By providing their compelling personal experiences of these difficult circumstances and their thoughtful reflections on surveys and observations to a world seeking answers, the authors of this volume are performing an act of leadership.

We thank the authors of this volume, who diligently took their chapters through several rounds of revisions. Thanks are also due to Gill Berchowitz, senior editor, and Sharon Rose, project editor, Ohio University Press; Susan Rhodes, director, HIV Training Institute, New York City Department of Health and formerly senior program officer of Population Communications International, New York, who provided detailed editorial comments on each chapter; Diane Ciekawy, professor of anthropology, Ohio University, and convenor of the IAC's

"HIV/AIDS and the African Child" conference; Matthew Adeyanju, professor of health sciences, and Gillian Ice, professor of social medicine, Ohio University, who reviewed the manuscripts submitted to this volume; Abdul Lamin and Acacia Nikoi, coordinators of the Institute of the African Child; and graduate students Li Wang, Pei-Wen Lee, and Ketan Chitnis of the College of Communication, Ohio University, who provided research assistance.

In the chapters that follow, we invite our readers to join the work of the Institute for the African Child in making childhood possible in Africa.

Afya njema!

Note

1. Emma Guest, *Children of AIDS: Africa's Orphan Crisis* (Pietermaritzburg: University of Natal Press, 2001).

Introduction

The Possibilities of African Leadership

W. Stephen Howard

"What shall we do?" is the refrain of Oliver Mtukudzi's popular song "Todii." This Zimbabwean master, who has reached his country's youth with his aptly named "Tuku music," wants an answer to his compelling question about the AIDS crisis. In its Declaration of Commitment on HIV/AIDS: Global Crisis—Global Action (June 2001) the United Nations General Assembly recognized the age-based dimensions of the pandemic and the need to focus on those most at risk, "particularly women and young people." During the UN debate, the *New York Times* published op-ed pieces by Secretary General Kofi Annan and the Mozambican prime minister, Pascoal Mocumbi. While the secretary general's column was appropriately diplomatic, the prime minister, perhaps hardened to the task by Mozambique's decades of poverty and war, made a courageous statement given the political climate:

> As a father, I fear for the lives of my own children and their teenage friends. Though they have secure families, education, and the information and support they need to avoid risky sex, too few of their peers do. As prime minister, I am horrified that we stand

to lose most of a generation, maybe two. The United Nations estimates that 37 percent of the 16-year-olds in my country will die of AIDS before they are 30. As a man, I know men's behavior must change, that we must raise boys differently, to have any hope of eradicating HIV and preventing the emergence of another such scourge.[1]

Africa's charge to modern leadership is the restoration of community. This is not a wistful desire for a (impossible or romantic) return to the static status quo ante, but rather a quest for the indigenous cultural, social, and political resources that have bound communities together. By *restoration* I mean a conscious effort to recognize the *processes* that may create secure and safe environments for Africa's children. These processes include communal vigilance, communal labor, and resources of kinship that in many cases promote a highly cooperative atmosphere. Rural people's knowledge—expertise derived from experience and communicated in an appropriate capacity-building mode—provides the curriculum for those acts of binding.[2] These community resources have been disrupted by colonialism, urban migration, industrialization, the collapse of agriculture, and political violence. The HIV/AIDS pandemic may be added to that list, particularly in the southern and eastern African nations most affected. Prime Minister Mocumbi's assertion of moral authority may be the first step required in establishing this type of leadership. He speaks as a leader who is a father, adding the respect of African family ties to that of state office.

The family provides some of the boundaries of childhood and youth in Africa, as it determines the movement from home to school to work, sets parameters for entry into society, and establishes the rules for marriage and the next generation. In the context of this volume, other age-related boundaries are the biological circumstances of birth and peri-natality, children's growth, and vulnerability to disease through malnutrition. Children's susceptibility to disease may be affected by social responsibilities that keep them out of school and other information pathways—family size, the child's place in the family constellation, participation in the family's decisions about schooling. The phenomenon of childhood itself can be seen as a window through which to view *all* other social interaction. A community's hopes and aspirations are embodied in their children; children present possibilities. They are the community's bright signal that, whatever else may be happening, life has important meaning. And the moment of childhood is fleeting, placing real urgency on the response to crises like HIV/AIDS. The dramatic question What shall we do? often galvanizes community action and in South Africa we see mass demonstrations in support of AIDS treatments and funerals of gigantic proportions. The engaged community leader responds, If we do not address this problem quickly, our future is much harder to imagine.

In looking at leadership, children, and HIV/AIDS in Africa, schooling is the most ubiquitous sector. The heavy emotional and economic investment that African communities make in securing education for their children is due to its perceived and actual role in social mobility. The grandmother in Sudan solemnly placing her hand on the head of her grandchild with the blessing, *In sha' Allah, t'itwazif* ("God willing, you'll be a bureaucrat") speaks volumes to community expectations of schooling. Prestige, stable employment, escape from rural poverty, and entrée to the resources associated with urban life are all part of the grandmother's wish that her grandchild have a better life than her own.

A major challenge to development in the postindependence period has been to increase the access of girls to schooling. That schools be part of the HIV/AIDS equation is consistent with their rootedness in the everyday life of Africa today.

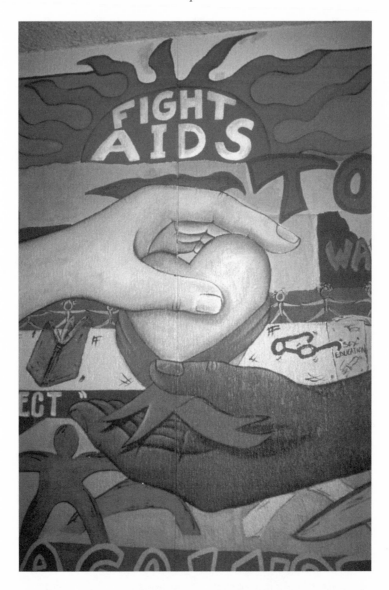

Fig. 0.1. An AIDS mural painted by adolescents at ML Sultan Technikon in South Africa to demonstrate their resolve in combating AIDS. Johns Hopkins University Center for Communication Programs. Photograph by Gary Lewis, JHU/CCP. Used with permission.

Every type of African community, both rural and urban, knows that education is about the most ubiquitous of infrastructure. Schools are the locus of local professionalism, and schoolteachers are often the most educated members of a community. Schools in Africa are centers of intercultural communication and contact, delivering a curriculum that tries to promote not only national unity but also global understanding. (I am always amazed at the precise recitation of European or American geography by African schoolchildren, in contrast to the fuzzy knowledge their American counterparts possess.)

Yet the geography of HIV/AIDS is a major threat to the continued progress of getting female children through Africa's schools. First, teachers are one of the largest professional groups infected with the AIDS virus in southern Africa—it has been reported that eighteen teachers were dying per month in Nairobi in 2001. This tragedy is a component of the deterioration of the early promise of teachers as rural development leaders in postindependence Africa. Second, when one or both parents in a family sicken or die, major responsibilities shift to daughters. Tsitsi Dangarembga's film *Everyone's Child* (1996) depicts a family of orphaned children as they decline into poverty and isolation with the death of parents from AIDS. Dangarembga is also the author of *Nervous Conditions*, a novel about girls and school in Zimbabwe. A study conducted with data from thirty-eight African countries revealed that the gross enrollment ratio for females decreased as HIV/AIDS infections rose.[3] With bitter irony it is reported that pupil-teacher ratios improve under these circumstances as well (i.e., class size is reduced).[4] The gross enrollment ratios for girls in the southern African countries were the highest on the continent prior to the HIV/AIDS devastation. Swaziland's education motto, *Umfundzo uze ufe* (You learn until the grave), takes on a new and ominous meaning, and the impact of the low status of women on their susceptibility to HIV infection is compounded in the case of girls.

Education is still crucial to African development, and girls' education can be a critical mitigating force to the HIV/AIDS threat, as it helps girls build individual identities and acquire the skills needed to support themselves in the community and beyond. The positive effect of girls' education on the wider community is even greater as educated girls become educated mothers who can contribute to household and community life with greater knowledge.

There has been serious growth in thought given to the role that school can play in changing community attitudes toward HIV/AIDS. Curricula are being developed by national ministries and international donor agencies that emphasize risk prevention behavior and stigma reduction, as well as simple means to help students and their families cope with illness. An overall theme of emphasizing girls' choices and ability to act is being worked out on paper and finding its way into donor discussions of education assistance, among other sectors of intervention.

The potency of this "education vaccine" against HIV/AIDS and other social ills depends on the whole support system for education, from infrastructure to teacher recruitment and preparation. The inoculation has not always taken and its lack of effectiveness disappoints parents and communities that have so heavily invested in education in the postindependence era. "Behavior change is possible," read the T-shirts distributed by a youth group dedicated to AIDS prevention in Swaziland, but operationalizing this earnest message is difficult, particularly if it is viewed not just as a personal credo but also as a campaign for major social reform. The impoverished status of schools and poorly trained teachers are the most devastating impediments to the vaccine's effectiveness. Schools have always been seen as the places that shape children's knowledge, attitudes, and practices. But teachers are not receiving the training or the materials that they need in order to share useful health information with their students. There are so many layers of leadership above the classroom teacher where directives and authority lie and yet action is often frozen when the subject is HIV/AIDS. Nevertheless in many cases, school is the locus that comes to planners' minds when pro-social messages must be delivered to children. The inclusion of trained youths as peer educators may reduce the burden on teaching staffs.

Indigenous nongovernmental organizations (NGOs), the second leadership sector in Africa, often take over the delivery of messages where schools cannot reach. These grassroots agencies, often focused on a single issue and modestly funded, contrast with the international NGO donor sector, an extension of bilateral and multilateral development assistance. One indigenous NGO is SWAN, a women's organization in northeast Nigeria trying to address HIV/AIDS in communities near four international borders. These women are designing and placing posters with local and culturally appropriate themes throughout the Bornu State region, in schools and in tailor shops that cater to women. And then there is South African gender commissioner Farid Esack, a leader of a courageous movement in Cape Town, Positive Muslims (HIV-positive members of the Muslim community). The organization has a special educational outreach to young people and provides moral and health support in a community where it is badly needed. The courage demonstrated by Positive Muslims, of course, is in the context of Islam, where the penalties and ostracism for sex outside marriage are particularly severe.

How do we account for the proliferation of NGOs that attend to children's issues, educational issues, HIV/AIDS issues? We could consider this phenomenon as the very active phase of *restoring community* (from my definition of leadership above). A combination of higher levels of education and lower levels of available government employment—which used to be the only objective of job-seeking graduates—accounts in part for the manifestations of leadership in these organizations. A related factor is the decline in the provision of government services, particularly in rural areas. The credos of self-reliance and civil society have long been on Africa's theoretical agenda and are now seeing implementation in the growing number of these NGOs.

Yet NGOs can target needs narrowly. Their small-scale operations are lean, mobile, and versatile, which has allowed many with educational and health themes, skills, and resources to pitch in with the HIV/AIDS prevention and treatment agenda. However, because NGOs are precariously funded, projects can be cut off in midstream, and due to their small scale their staff may lack the knowledge needed in a complex area like the prevention and treatment of HIV/AIDS. The current trend toward partnerships between these local NGOs and multilateral or bilateral agencies is important as networks and multisectoral approaches are key in the war on HIV/AIDS. But in encouraging these partnerships we must be careful that the purpose of having locally based agencies addressing local needs is not defeated. The potential of these organizations to grow local leadership can be encouraged, and the element of children's participation is easier to promote with local groups. Families and other individuals known to children play a special role in easing children into civil society, and there are many organizations that specialize in promoting children as research assistants, monitors of community conditions (e.g., sanitation and safety), and participants in intergenerational development teams. In the cases of children in refugee situations and displacement, the mobility of resources in the larger organizations is probably a better choice for service delivery.

Finally, in this tour of the possibilities of child-centered leadership for HIV/AIDS prevention and treatment in Africa, it is important to mention the Institute for the African Child at

Ohio University, the sponsor of this publication. The institute was founded in 1998 to help both medical and health specialists and social scientists and humanists crack each other's secret codes for research and service on issues related to Africa's children. The academic field of African studies has conventionally excluded the medical and professional fields from its deliberations, but no single discipline has all the answers to these most complex of human issues. The Institute for the African Child has joined the foundational African studies fields in the social sciences and humanities with interested faculty in communication, education, health and human services, and osteopathic medicine in common purpose. The institute's perspective covers the niche of childhood studies, but childhood is also intimately attached to the African mother, the family, community, national policy, and continental trends. In the chapters that follow are a variety of perspectives from African societies and institutions, selected to demonstrate the child-centric actions that are possible in the face of this worldwide public health disaster.

As the world asks about what to do about the many threats to its security, a foundation of that security—the health of our children—is unstable. We seek new meanings with this volume, with the assumption that children experience the world in a qualitatively different way from adults. Their experiences of health and ill-health, care giving and receiving, messages delivered and received, are gaps in our understanding of the swath AIDS is cutting through African societies. Probing those experiences may offer insights as to how childhood in Africa may remain a joyful possibility.

Notes

1. *New York Times*, June 29, 2001, A29.

2. Robert Chambers, *Rural Development, Putting the Last First* (Essex, UK: Longman, 1983).

3. Gross enrollment ratio (GER) is the total number of students enrolling in school, regardless of age, expressed as a percentage of the official school age population.

4. USAID, "Colloquium on HIV/AIDS and Girls' Education" (2000): 10.

Section 1

VULNERABILITY

1

AIDS, Orphans, and the
Future of Democracy in Africa

Amy S. Patterson

Nengomasha Willard teaches eleven- and twelve-year-olds in rural Zimbabwe. Fifteen of his forty-two pupils have lost one or both of their parents to AIDS. He is worried about the impact of such a loss on all fifteen students, but particularly on one young boy who lost his father and then, at his mother's funeral, cried constantly. Willard says the child does not want to participate in school or youth activities. "He just wants to be alone."[1]

In Kenya, a woman whose sister died of AIDS, and who cares for her own children and her sister's children, describes how her sister was treated after she became a widow: "After my sister's husband died, she turned to her in-laws for help, but they told her to move from the house. She sold vegetables to make money and stayed outside the property much of the time. They treated her this way because of the property, which they wanted. She became a useless person to them, the same as the children."[2]

Because of the high rate of HIV/AIDS in Bahir Dar, Ethiopia, children as young as eight are taking care of siblings. They face ostracism from the community, exclusion from schools and living areas, and loneliness. One orphaned head of household said, "Neighbors do not want us to join them . . . because we are identified as children whose parents died of HIV/AIDS and there is a rumor that we are infected with the virus. . . . People talk about us negatively everywhere, and we feel ashamed."[3]

These brief examples illustrate the great personal, economic, and social impact of HIV/AIDS on individuals and families. Yet, these stories also show that AIDS (and its social and economic implications) may cause individuals to change how they view themselves within the community. Those left behind after relatives die of AIDS may withdraw from the community, become worthless in the eyes of others, or feel ashamed because they are excluded from communal activities. As AIDS shapes the relationships that people have with their communities, individuals then change their view of their rights and responsibilities as citizens within the political realm. These new forms of political identity can influence how individuals participate in politics.

Most political scientists have neglected the intersection of politics and AIDS in Africa.[4] However, AIDS influences political actions because it constrains state resources, changes the nature of political communities, and reconfigures how individuals view their rights and responsibilities within those communities. Examining the impact of AIDS on individual citizens and political communities is crucial, since Africa experienced a wave of democratization in the 1990s. Because individuals, either alone or through the organization of civil society, played a key role in facilitating democracy in many African states, it is important to understand how AIDS influences individual notions of citizenship.[5]

This chapter investigates how one consequence of AIDS—the increased number of African orphans—may affect Africa's democratization process. This work defines an AIDS orphan as any child under the age of fifteen who has lost one or both parents to AIDS.[6] How might AIDS shape the ability of these young people to learn democratic values, such as participation, tolerance, compromise, accountability, transparency, and political efficacy?

Political Socialization and Democracy in Africa

Democratization efforts in Africa began in 1990 with the emergence of a sovereign national conference in Benin and the release of Nelson Mandela in South Africa. Prior to 1990 most African regimes were one-party states (e.g., Kenya and Tanzania), military regimes (e.g., Ghana and Nigeria), or semi-democracies that controlled the electoral process (e.g., Botswana and Senegal). By 1997, however, only Nigeria, Somalia, Swaziland, and Zaire had not held a competitive multiparty election at the national level.[7] On one hand, elections have become a simplistic measure of democracy and a vehicle through which African states have gained international legitimacy.[8] On the other hand, even with flawed elections, the military has returned to power in only four countries that underwent democratic liberalization in the early 1990s, and a general acceptance of the value of elections has emerged.[9] Africa has also experienced the rise of independent news media and nongovernmental organizations (NGOs)[10] that foster democratic participation, and more African states now protect civil and political liberties than before 1990.[11]

I define a democracy as a system in which individuals participate, either directly or indirectly, in decision making; use various methods to hold leaders accountable for their actions; and exhibit specific values, such as tolerance and a willingness to compromise and build consensus.[12] Political scientists know that these attitudes and behaviors are learned through the life-long, uncritical, and casual process of political socialization.[13] While the period between fourteen and twenty-five years of age is believed to be especially important for the development of political attitudes,[14] I argue that the socialization of African children under the age of fourteen should not be ignored.[15] Many African preadolescents are put into adult situations, such as working for the family, caring for other children, or fighting in wars. These adult responsibilities may cause African youth to become more politically aware at a younger age than their counterparts in industrial societies.

The family, the community, peers, religious organizations, the media, and educational institutions influence political attitudes. Although scholars no longer view the family to be the most durable influence on political attitudes, the family has the earliest impact on a child's attitudinal development.[16] As Jean Whyte discovered for Northern Irish youth, a child's family situation may serve as a lens through which politics is viewed.[17] Similarly, because the African family shapes communities, power relationships, and property ownership, it plays an important socializing function.[18] Schools also facilitate socialization because they teach students to respect authority, cooperate with others, and participate as citizens.[19] Structured academic activities that encourage students to critically discuss political issues can foster participation, accountability, and democratic values.[20] Likewise, school-affiliated and community groups, such as voluntary associations and service clubs, provide an opportunity for youth to incorporate civic involvement into their identity during key points in their lives. As youth learn the basic roles and processes of organizations, they also learn about political discourse, the coordination of multiple perspectives, and the interdependence of actions.[21] These educational experiences may be crucial for encouraging democratic values in societies that have recently undergone democratic transitions.[22]

The process of political socialization does not always encourage individuals to support the status quo. Three examples illustrate how political, economic, and social upheavals can create changes in political attitudes among youth or adults. First, in postindustrial societies, the lack of entry-level jobs and the high cost of education have left many youth without a clear social niche. This phenomenon has contributed to a decline in youth political participation,[23] an increase in youth depression and suicide,[24] and a culture of youth violence in some urban areas.[25] Second, youth who were socialized during South Africa's transition from apartheid tend to be more concerned about violence and the country's future and less trusting of the state.[26] Third, structural adjustment economic policies have led to new attitudes about citizenship rights and responsibilities in Senegalese village associations.[27]

Socialization literature raises numerous questions about the role of AIDS orphans in African politics. How will traditional agents of socialization, and new types of socialization experiences that emerge because of AIDS, affect the political attitudes of AIDS orphans? I now turn my attention to these questions.

AIDS Orphans and Africa's Political Future

Even before the death of a family member, AIDS places extreme pressure on the family and community.[28] Children may live with long periods of uncertainty and periods of crisis as they watch parents slowly become sicker and more incapacitated. Communities may suffer from the loss of leaders, taxpayers, and producers, and social institutions may be unable to meet rising demands for health and social services.[29] These changes in family and community can have a profound impact on political socialization and the development of citizenship.

AIDS and Political Socialization in the Family

The impact of AIDS on children differs, depending on which family member is infected. The death of a father from AIDS often leads to crises over family income and inheritance. In such cases, it is not uncommon for property to revert back to the husband's family and for the mother and her children to be forced to return to her own family.[30] Yet, this extended family support is not always available for women living in urban areas far from their rural families. In such cases, women may earn money through informal businesses, including prostitution.[31] Children in these female-headed households are more likely to be malnourished, to lack educational opportunities, and to be unhealthy. Difficult working conditions and the strain of financial obligations may accelerate the health decline of an HIV-positive mother who contracted the disease from her husband.[32] Children whose mothers die from AIDS face the psychological trauma of losing their primary caregiver. Child neglect and abandonment by fathers after the death of a mother have been documented in several African countries.[33]

Within the context of these changes, how can the family influence the political socialization of children? First, in most African societies men dominate the public realm of politics.[34] Men disproportionately serve as local councilors, village elders, and elected officials. Men also are more likely to have the time, energy, and confidence to participate in public debates on politics.[35] If children lose a father to AIDS, they may have fewer opportunities to observe the public role that citizens play in politics. These children may have less exposure to political conversations in the home or be less aware of the role of adults in political activities such as elections or village meetings.

The absence of politically active men may give women the opportunity to fill this vacuum and become political actors in public venues. Yet, a second implication of AIDS for orphans' socialization is that women may not have time for political activities. If single women must work, care for children, and provide for the household, they may have little time or energy for political involvement.[36] The extra demands that social and economic changes in the family place on women because of AIDS may also mean they cannot participate in traditional women's activities, such as rotating-credit societies or state-affiliated development projects. If children do not observe their mothers model participation by attending group meetings or working on cooperative projects, children may get the message that participation in such communal activities is not important.

Third, because AIDS deaths may lead to conflicts in families over the inheritance of property, children may learn divisive attitudes, rather than democratic values such as compromise, tolerance, and conflict resolution. Instead of learning how to work with others to build consensus, children may view their communities and families as arenas of division. One child in Kenya explains what happened after her parents both died of AIDS: "My father's relatives said that the property didn't go with me and my sister, and they said go back to Nairobi to what you're used to."[37] This story, and the case of the Kenyan woman who lost her property (related above), illustrate how children may perceive decisions about resources to be winner-take-all, instead of based on compromise. Finally, if families deny property to children or their mothers, AIDS orphans may deduce that the political system does not protect their interests. Children often have little standing in the legal realm. They are uninformed about laws that may exist to protect their rights, and it is difficult for them to acquire legal representation.[38] Because of their exclusion from the legal realm, children's political efficacy and political trust may be greatly eroded.

Because of the spread of HIV—the virus that causes AIDS—most AIDS orphans today who have lost both parents are cared for by extended family members, particularly maternal grandmothers who are widows.[39] Lacking resources, educational skills, and the safety net that they had expected in their old age, these grandmothers are often unable to provide for orphaned children socially or economically. Children in these households may lack access to adequate food, shelter, and health care.[40] In addition to these deficiencies, the stresses put on the family through new institutional arrangements can have a long-term psychological impact on children.[41]

This pattern of extended-family care also may influence how and what children learn about the political realm. First, children who are cared for by widowed grandmothers may not have much exposure to male individuals acting in public politics. While some grandmothers may fill the political void created by younger male AIDS casualties, it is likely that the time, energy, and financial strains on older caregivers will limit their ability to participate in political activities. Second, because they may not form strong bonds with the community of their extended family,[42] orphaned children may have a decreased sense of communal obligation, and they may feel somewhat alienated from local politics.[43] Third, as the case of the children in Ethiopia illustrates, children who have parents who died of AIDS often experience shame and rejection by their community or peers.[44] This rejection may reinforce the feeling that AIDS orphans are not citizens of the community and that their participation in communal endeavors is not welcome. Finally, since discrimination may limit access to health, education, and social services, AIDS orphans may learn that politics and political benefits are exclusive.[45] This view may cause political and social alienation, apathy, and low political efficacy.

AIDS and Political Socialization in Schools

AIDS has greatly affected Africa's educational system. First, because AIDS has had a disproportionate impact on educated workers such as teachers, AIDS orphans (and children in general) will have fewer opportunities for good, consistent educational experiences. For example, it is estimated that 30 percent of teachers in Malawi and Zambia are HIV positive.[46] This percentage will certainly increase as companies that lose workers to AIDS woo teachers as replacements, offering salaries that educational institutions cannot match.[47] Alan Whiteside, an AIDS researcher at the University of Natal, says, "Teachers who fall sick will not all be replaced, and you can never replicate a week or a term of teaching in the life of a child."[48] The educational process may become much more haphazard, as HIV-positive teachers become ill and cannot attend classes or as schools lie vacant waiting for teacher replacements.

Moreover, AIDS has caused governments to divert funds from education to health care in order to care for the rising number of AIDS patients. In countries such as Malawi, Zimbabwe, and Rwanda, over 50 percent of government health spending is used for AIDS care.[49] The World Bank estimates that the money used to treat one AIDS patient with the so-called drug cocktail would keep four hundred children in school for a year.[50] While the public demands health services, the opportunity cost of not adequately educating future generations can be quite high. Because education increases an individual's earning power, affects the age when women will marry and have children, and influences health care decisions, AIDS spending for Africa's educational system can greatly impede Africa's development.[51]

Finally, AIDS orphans have less exposure to the benefits of the educational system because they are less likely to attend school.[52] Even before they become orphans, children (especially girls) may be forced to leave school to care for younger siblings and ill family members or to earn money for the family. After a parent's death, orphans may leave school to work to supplement the extended family's income. Overburdened with children and limited in educational and employment skills, older caregivers also may lack the financial resources to pay for school fees.[53] Orphans may be denied access to education, especially if parents, students, and teachers erroneously fear that these children may spread AIDS to others.

These trends in education can have an impact on the process of political socialization. Education enables people to better understand political issues and to feel confident about participating in politics.[54] Education gives individuals the needed critical thinking and communication skills to influence policymakers and to creatively address community problems. Further, activities associated with educational institutions, such as service clubs or volunteer groups, teach young people important democratic values such as participation, compromise, tolerance, and consensus building. If Africa's educational systems deteriorate because of a shortage of teachers and lack of state investment, young people will have fewer opportunities to develop a political identity within a safe and constructive environment. If governments are unable to provide educational opportunities, young people may get the impression that they are a low priority in government policymaking. Additionally, if AIDS orphans are less likely to attend school, they will not be exposed to certain positive socializing experiences. Lower rates of political participation and low political efficacy may result.

Additionally, teachers are high-status members of the community, who are valued because of the ways that they model behavior, hard work, and community norms. Teachers can play a unique role for students without parents, encouraging orphans to excel in school and to participate in school activities. The shortage of teachers will mean that there are fewer adults who can influence the social, political, and educational development of Africa's young people, especially its orphans. The outcome may be that "[w]e face a generation growing up that is disaffected, unskilled, and desocialized because of AIDS."[55]

AIDS Orphans, Socialization, and Political Uncertainty

Family, economic, and educational uncertainties affect all AIDS orphans, especially those who live in child-headed households. Though most AIDS orphans are cared for by extended family members, there has been an increase in child-headed households, especially in urban areas.[56] There are several implications for the increasing numbers of AIDS orphans living without adult supervision. First, these orphans often must engage in dangerous labor, such as prostitution and theft.[57] Such activities put them at a higher risk for contracting HIV. This risk is apparent for young women aged fifteen to nineteen, for whom the HIV infection rate is six times that of their male counterparts.[58] Second, because children need physical and emotional security if they are to become happy and healthy adults, AIDS orphans living on their own are significantly more likely to be psychologically depressed.[59] Depression can make them more susceptible to suicide and drug use. In Malawi tens of thousands of orphans have turned to begging and drugs.[60]

Third, because of economic difficulties, drug use, and the lack of adult supervision, AIDS orphans may be more inclined to turn to crime. South African crime researcher Martin Schönteich says, "In a decade's time every fourth South African will be between 15 and 24 years of age. It is in this age group where people's propensity to commit crime is at its highest. At about the same time there will be a boom in South Africa's orphan population as the AIDS epidemic takes its toll."[61] Already strained by rising health costs, government budgets may be unable to address the increasing cost of crime. Additionally, children who grow up in an atmosphere of crime and violence may become desensitized to the human cost of violent actions and accept such activities as normal. These children may learn that problems are solved through force, not dialogue, compromise, negotiation, and consensus building. Youth socialized in cultures of violence are more likely to exhibit aggressive behavior later in life.[62] Finally, without a family, village, or neighborhood to shape their identity, orphans are more vulnerable to manipulation by adults. Orphans may turn to older adults for love, affirmation, and care; and adults may capitalize on the disenfranchisement that orphans feel.[63]

There are three ways that the socialization experiences of these young people may hamper Africa's democratic future. First, AIDS orphans will swell the already high numbers of urban, unemployed youth. These urban young people have contributed to the increased political violence surrounding African elections, strikes, and protests. For example, in the March 2002 presidential election in Zimbabwe the ruling party sought to prevent the opposition from freely competing in the election. Youth supporting President Robert Mugabe were mobilized into militia groups called Taliban, which set up temporary camps outside voting places to antagonize election observers and intimidate opposition supporters.[64] In this context, *taliban*—the Arabic term for students, the base of support of the former Afghan regime—connotes disaffected young people who are easily mobilized for violence by adults and who may be ruthless in their (the students') revolutionary zeal. The presence of a large number of unemployed youth who feel they have few economic and social options made it easy to mobilize them to do the party's dirty work. As AIDS decreases economic development, income-generating opportunities, and government resources, individuals may scramble for the few economic resources that the state controls, and AIDS orphans may be incorporated into increasingly violent and desperate political competition.[65]

Second, the U.S. Central Intelligence Agency predicts that the growing number of AIDS orphans will exacerbate the pervasive use of child soldiers in African conflicts.[66] Currently there are over 120,000 child soldiers fighting in twelve different African countries. Though some of these children were abducted into armed conflict, others feel they have no other option but military service. As the number of AIDS orphans increases, the number of disaffected and impoverished youth who see military service as a way to gain community and material benefits will increase.[67] Because of their dire material situation, and because of their need to be accepted, AIDS orphans also may be more likely to participate in dangerous military activities, such as intelligence work and bombing missions.[68] For example, hundreds of former child soldiers in Liberia returned to military service after President Charles Taylor declared a state of emergency in March 2002. These young ex-combatants had no food, shelter, or employment and thus felt they had little choice but to join the army again.[69]

Child soldiers are socialized into a culture of violence that makes them less likely to question their actions and more likely to use force to achieve their goals. Interviews with civilians in Sierra Leone illustrate the inability of these young people to empathize, compromise, or care for others. One adult victim of child soldiers said, "We feared them [the young rebels]. They were cruel and hard hearted; even more than the adults. They don't know what is sympathy; what is good and bad. If you beg an older one you may convince him to spare you, but the younger ones, they don't know what is sympathy, what is mercy. Those who have been rebels for so long have never learned it."[70] Illustrating how young rebels view political conflict to be a zero-sum game with no restraints, another civilian repeated what a child soldier had said to him, "We can do anything we want in Freetown. We don't have mothers; we don't have fathers. We can do anything we want."[71] The political attitudes that emerge from these socialization experiences will surely detract from Africa's democratization process.[72]

A third way that the rise of AIDS orphans may hamper African democratization is through the recruitment of these children into terrorist networks. Though terrorists traditionally have been young adults in their twenties with some education, research indicates that in recent years, more terrorists are increasingly younger, less educated, and from desperate economic situations.[73] In the Middle East, the Philippines, Sri Lanka, and Colombia, teenagers, some as young as twelve, have perpetrated terrorist attacks.[74] Recognizing the potentially explosive nature of this situation, Senator Joseph Biden, former chair of the U.S. Senate Committee on Foreign Relations, has said that if the AIDS pandemic is not reversed, "We will have much more than a health problem; we will have a security problem" because unstable countries with large numbers of disaffected youth "are susceptible to the future bin Ladens of the world."[75]

Policy Recommendations for International Donors and NGOs

Several policy prescriptions follow from the various roles that AIDS orphans may play in Africa's political future. It goes without saying that the basic survival needs of AIDS orphans must be met. Currently, most NGOs and international donors[76] seek to achieve this goal by providing income-generating opportunities for extended family members or monetary grants during crucial times.[77] Donors and NGOs should continue these efforts and should devote more resources to them. If children's basic needs are not met, AIDS orphans will be even more likely to turn to destructive activities. Yet if donors and NGOs hope to foster citizenship among these young people, they must go beyond just meeting orphans' basic needs.

Develop Positive Role Models

Young people must have positive role models who can demonstrate important democratic values, such as participation, empathy, and tolerance. Because AIDS changes community and family structures, these adult role models may come in new forms. For example, rather than children looking to fathers, village chiefs, or schoolteachers to model participation and consensus building, they may look to the new associations that have formed around the issue of AIDS. Groups of widows, youth organizations, burial societies, and adult groups organized to care for orphans can provide such role models.

Model Democracy through Disclosure

The National Community of Women Living with HIV/AIDS (NACWOLA) was created in 1992 by a small group of HIV-positive Ugandan women. These women sought a way to disclose their health status to their children, knowing that secrecy would be psychologically and emotionally destructive. The group provides peer support for children and families affected by HIV, and it gives children a safe place in which to discuss the difficulties they face having HIV-positive parents. The women in the organization also work to provide services such as vocational training for children and succession planning for families. By cooperating to make decisions for children, by treating HIV-positive parents with dignity and respect, and by helping adults to be open with their children about their health, the members of this organization model important democratic values such as participation, tolerance, and transparency.[78]

Encourage Education

AIDS orphans must be educated, because education opens the door to future economic opportunities and instills confidence and critical-thinking skills. Given the resource constraints that orphans and their caregivers face, donors must provide free education, books, and supplies. Donors and NGOs also need to help families replace the revenue lost when children attend school and do not work. In some communities, volunteer schools have condensed a curriculum or rearranged school schedules to better accommodate children and their families.[79] Additionally, African governments, with the help of donor nations, must train more teachers, so that AIDS does not decimate their numbers. In the short run, donors can address the teacher shortage through volunteer programs such as the U.S. Peace Corps or UN volunteers. Donors can also address the teacher shortage by providing funds to improve the salaries that teachers receive. This policy may encourage teachers to stay in the educational profession, instead of working for industry. Donors must focus efforts on educational institutions because teachers and schools play such a big role in developing citizenship.

Local communities also can play a large role in providing educational opportunities for orphans. For example, in Kitwe, Zambia, community members have lobbied the local school management committee to waive the fees for orphans and other vulnerable children in the village. Although this has had a negative impact on the school's operating budget, fees have been waived for almost one-third of the school's fifteen hundred students. Community-initiated income projects have also been used in the village to raise money to pay the school fees for orphans.[80] Such efforts enable orphans to remain in school and demonstrate to these children that they are valued within the community. Such intangible lessons contribute to developing a sense of citizenship among these young people.

Develop Avenues to Promote Democratic Values among Youth

Young people must be given the opportunity to shape AIDS policies. The development of a political identity requires that individuals have the opportunity to be serious participants in making decisions, especially about issues that affect them directly. AIDS orphans and other vulnerable children must be invited to share their stories and provide their ideas about how donors can meet their needs, though NGOs and donors must be careful not to single out these children or to facilitate their ostracism in the community.

All local decision-making bodies that address AIDS issues should include youth representatives and should value their participation. At times, including youth in decision making may appear to challenge the power of older people in African society. Yet youth participation is essential because it leads to more effective AIDS programs and because it enables young people to practice compromise, negotiation, and leadership. Further, as young people work with NGOs and donors to make decisions about such programs, they develop political efficacy.

Teach Democracy through Peer Interactions

The Zambia Morehouse/YWCA out-of-school project illustrates how a community program can teach important democratic values and build youth efficacy while also countering AIDS. In cooperation with the Morehouse University School of Medicine, YWCA program workers select and train teens that are at risk of contracting HIV/AIDS to serve as volunteer peer outreach workers (POWs) in their communities. POWs provide information, counseling, and instruction in decision making, using the methods of large-group presentations, small-group discussions, and one-on-one visits with youth clients. POWs work together with program staff to decide which methods to incorporate and which strategies to use in targeting various clients.

Several positive outcomes of the peer educator program have emerged. POWs have discovered how important it is to understand their peers. These skills are not only important for the success of the AIDS education program but also are needed for consensus building in any community. Likewise, POWs have learned how to model to their peers the importance of community involvement. By giving their time and by risking social ostracism because they talk about AIDS, these young people demonstrate concern for the community's improvement, a willingness to work with others, and the responsibilities of citizenship. POWs also develop a sense of efficacy, in that they believe they can shape the future of their communities. One POW reported, "At times you share an idea with a friend and later discover that person accepted the idea. You see the change. It just gives self-pride, self-satisfaction. It's also beneficial because you turn out to be a role model."[81] The sense of efficacy that POWs develop is reinforced by the fact that the community is very involved in the program. Adult POWs help to ensure that parents of targeted youth and other adults in the community are educated about HIV/AIDS. Moreover, local religious leaders publicly support the work of adult and youth POWs. The important services that these at-risk youth perform in their communities have helped them develop a sense of the rights and responsibilities of citizenship.[82]

Recognize the Rights of Young People and Teach Them about Their Rights

In order to limit political alienation and develop political efficacy, HIV-positive African youth must perceive that the political system seeks to meet their needs and the needs of all those with HIV and AIDS. In both domestic and international political spheres, AIDS orphans have few advocates.[83] When young people believe that political leaders do not care about them, they may be more likely to participate in activities against the system.[84] The rights of children to information, education, inheritance, and safety must not only be acknowledged through the passage of national legislation and international resolutions, but these rights must be strictly enforced.[85] Young people need to be informed of their rights and the ways that local, national, and international institutions protect those rights. For example, UNICEF bases its AIDS-prevention programs on the belief that young people have the right to the knowledge and skills that reduce their vulnerability.[86] Similarly, Zambia's Children in Need Network strives to increase policymakers' awareness of the rights of orphans and vulnerable children and lobbies the government for policies that will benefit such children.[87] When young people better understand their rights and have the confidence and skills to exercise those rights, they can better contribute to fighting AIDS and to fostering African democracy.

No one knows exactly what the impact of AIDS will be on Africa's political future. Yet, because of the high personal, family, community, social, and economic costs of the pandemic, it would be naïve to assume that AIDS will not influence the realm of politics as well. One way that AIDS may change the future of the continent is by shaping the political attitudes and behaviors of Africa's future citizens, millions of whom will be AIDS orphans.

Given the uncertainty of Africa's political future, international donors, governments, NGOs, community activists, and other adults in positions of power must recognize that AIDS orphans are vulnerable, fragile, and in need of care, love, and acceptance. While AIDS challenges individuals and communities, it also provides opportunities for young people and adults to model care, participation, honesty, and acceptance through newly formed associations and programs designed to address the pandemic. These new means of fostering citizenship among Africa's young people must be encouraged. Otherwise, sustaining Africa's nascent democracies will be difficult.

Notes

1. *The Village Voice*, November 3–9, 1999.

2. Human Rights Watch, "In the Shadow of Death: HIV/AIDS and Children's Rights in Kenya," *Human Rights Watch Report* 13, 4 (2001): 18.

3. Marta Segu and Sergut Wolde-Yohannes, "A Mounting Crisis: Children Orphaned by HIV/AIDS in Semiurban Ethiopia," *Orphan Alert: International Perspectives on Children Left Behind by HIV/AIDS*, formerly at <http://www.fxb.org>, n.d.

4. Catherine Boone and Jake Batsell, "Politics and AIDS in Africa: Research Agendas in Political Science and International Relations," <http://iupjournals.org/africatoday/aft48-2.html>, 2001.

5. Larry Diamond and Marc Plattner, ed., *Democratization in Africa* (Baltimore: Johns Hopkins University Press, 1999).

6. Susan Hunter and John Williamson, "Children on the Brink: Strategies to Support Children Isolated by HIV/AIDS" (report for USAID, Washington, 1997). Different organizations define orphanhood in various ways. UNAIDS, for example, defines an orphan as any child under fifteen who has lost his or her mother or both parents (UNAIDS 2001). I use the more inclusive definition because loss of either parent to AIDS can cause psychological, economic, and emotional trauma to a child.

7. Michael Bratton, "Second Elections in Africa," in *Democratization in Africa*, ed. Larry Diamond and Marc Plattner (Baltimore: Johns Hopkins University Press, 1999), 18–33.

8. Richard Joseph, "Africa, 1990–1997: From Abertura to Closure," in *Democratization in Africa*, ed. Larry Diamond and Marc Plattner (Baltimore: Johns Hopkins University Press, 1999), 3–17.

9. Bratton, "Second Elections in Africa." These countries are Burundi, Congo-Brazzaville, Niger, and Sierra Leone. Some of these countries, such as Sierra Leone, have held multiparty elections since the military takeovers.

10. When I use the term NGO, I refer to indigenous NGOs.

11. E. Gyimah-Boadi, "The Rebirth of African Liberalism," in *Democratization in Africa*, ed. Larry Diamond and Marc Plattner (Baltimore: Johns Hopkins University Press, 1999), 34–47; Freedom House, "Freedom in the World 2002: The Democracy Gap," <http://www.freedomhouse.org/research/survey2002.htm>, 2002; Diamond and Plattner, *Democratization in Africa*. In 2002, Freedom

House classified nine African countries as *free*, twenty-five countries as *partly free*, and nineteen as *not free*. A country is free if it receives a score of 1–3 on a combined measure of political rights and civil liberties, partly free if the score is 3.5–5, and not free if the score is 5.5–7. For both political rights and civil liberties, countries are rated on a seven-point scale, with one representing the most free and seven representing the least free. Political rights include the right to form parties that represent a range of voter choices and that have leaders who can compete for office. Civil liberties include religious, ethnic, economic, linguistic, and gender rights; freedom of the press; and freedom of association. While these numbers indicate that democracy has not been fully consolidated in Africa, they are an improvement from 1989, when only three countries were rated as free, eleven partly free, and thirty-three not free. (Fewer countries were assessed in 1989 because Freedom House did not then include Namibia, Eritrea, and four North African countries in its analysis.)

12. Naomi Chazan, "Africa's Democratic Challenge," *World Policy Journal* 9, 2 (1993): 279–307; Larry Diamond, *Political Culture and Democracy in Developing Countries* (Boulder: Lynne Rienner, 1993); Amy Patterson, "Participation and Democracy at the Grassroots: A Study of Development Associations in Rural Senegal" (Ph.D. diss., Indiana University, 1996); Robert Putnam, *Making Democracy Work* (Princeton: Princeton University Press, 1993). These means of holding leaders accountable could include public actions, such as elections or derogatory songs, or more private methods, such as gossip.

13. Pamela Conover, "Political Socialization: Where's the Politics?" in *Political Science: Looking to the Future*, 4 volumes, ed. William Crotty (Evanston: Northwestern University Press, 1991), 3: 125–52.

14. Richard Niemi and Mary Hepburn, "The Rebirth of Political Socialization," *Perspectives on Political Science* 24, 1 (1995): 7–16.

15. Niemi and Hepburn report that many political scientists do not examine the political socialization of youth below the age of fourteen because political concepts are too complicated for these youth. Most political scientists also assume that youth below the age of fourteen cannot reason consequentially, understand the long-range implications of various courses of action, or deduce specific choices from general principles. Most also lack an interest in politics. Niemi and Hepburn, "Rebirth."

16. M. Kent Jennings and Richard Niemi, "The Transmission of Political Values from Parent to Child," in *Socialization to Politics: A*

Reader, ed. Jack Dennis (New York: Wiley, 1973), 3–17; Fred Greenstein, *Children and Politics* (New Haven: Yale University Press, 1965); Herbert Hyman, *Political Socialization: A Study of the Psychology of Political Behavior* (New York: Free Press, 1959).

17. Jean Whyte, "Young Citizens in Changing Times: Catholics and Protestants in Northern Ireland," *Journal of Social Issues* 54, 2 (1998): 603–20.

18. Brian Siegel, "Family and Kinship," in *Understanding Contemporary Africa*, ed. April Gordon and Donald Gordon (Boulder: Westview Press, 1996), 221–48.

19. David Koff, George von der Muhll, and Kenneth Prewitt, "Political Socialization in Three East African Countries: A Comparative Analysis," in *Socialization to Politics: A Reader*, ed. Jack Dennis (New York: Wiley, 1973), 231–56.

20. Roxanna Morduchowicz, Edgardo Catterberg, Richard Niemi, and Frank Bell, "Teaching Political Information and Democratic Values in a New Democracy: An Argentine Experiment," *Comparative Politics* 28, 4 (1996): 465–76; Niemi and Hepburn, "Rebirth of Political Socialization."

21. James Youniss, Jeff McLellan, and Miranda Yates, "What We Know about Engendering Civic Identity," *American Behavioral Scientist* 40, 5 (1997): 620–31.

22. Gyorgy Csepeli, *From Subject to Citizen* (Budapest: Hungarian Center for Political Education, 1994); Morduchowicz et al., "Teaching Political Information."

23. Harwood Group, *College Students Talk Politics* (Dayton: Kettering Foundation, 1993).

24. James Cote and Anton Allahar, *Generation on Hold: Coming of Age in the Late Twentieth Century* (New York: New York University Press, 1995).

25. Constance Flanagan and Lonnie Sherrod, "Youth Political Development: An Introduction," *Journal of Social Issues* 54, 3 (1998): 447–56.

26. Gillian Finchilescu and Andrew Dawes, "Catapulted into Democracy: South African Adolescents' Sociopolitical Orientations Following Rapid Social Change," *Journal of Social Issues* 54, 3 (1998): 563–83.

27. Amy Patterson, "The Dynamic Nature of Citizenship and Participation: Lessons from Three Rural Senegalese Case Studies," *Africa Today* 46, 1 (1999): 2–27.

28. UNICEF, "Children Orphaned by AIDS: Front-Line Responses from Eastern and Southern Africa," <http://www.unicef.org/pubsgen/aids>, 2000.

29. Meredith Turshen, "The Political Ecology of AIDS in Africa," in *The Political Economy of AIDS*, ed. Merrill Singer (Amityville, N.Y.: Baywood Publishing, 1998), 169–84.

30. Nigel Hall, ed., *Family Coping and AIDS in Zimbabwe: A Study* (Harare: University of Zimbabwe, 1994).

31. Brooke Grundfest Schoepf, "AIDS, Gender, and Sexuality during Africa's Economic Crisis," in *African Feminism: The Politics of Survival in Sub-Saharan Africa*, ed. Gwendolyn Mikell (Philadelphia: University of Pennsylvania Press, 1997), 310–32; Nancy Romero-Daza and David Himelgreen, "More than Money for Your Labor: Migration and the Political Economy of AIDS in Lesotho," in *The Political Economy of AIDS*, ed. Merrill Singer (Amityville, N.Y.: Baywood Publishing, 1998), 185–204.

32. *Village Voice*, December 1–7, 1999.

33. Hall, *Family Coping*; UNAIDS, UNICEF, and BLCA, "Call to Action for 'Children Left Behind' by AIDS" (report for UNICEF, New York, 1999); G. Foster, C. Makufa, R. Drew, S. Mashumba, and S. Kambeu, "Perceptions of Children and Community Members Concerning the Circumstances of Orphans in Rural Zimbabwe," *AIDS Care* 9, 4 (1997): 391–405.

34. This does not mean that women in African societies play no role in politics. Rather, women have tended to dominate the realm of private discussions and to use private actions to shape political decisions. Linda Beck, "Democratization and the 'Hidden Public': The Impact of Patronage Politics on Senegalese Women," *Comparative Politics* 35, 2 (2003): 147–71; Aili Mari Tripp, "Gender, Political Participation, and the Transformation of Associational Life in Uganda and Tanzania," *African Studies Review* 37, 1 (1994): 107–31; Janet MacGaffey, "Civil Society in Zaire: Hidden Resistance and the Use of Personal Ties in Class Struggle," in *Civil Society and the State in Africa*, ed. John Harbeson, Donald Rothchild, and Naomi Chazan (Boulder: Lynne Rienner, 1994), 169–89; Patterson, "Participation and Democracy."

35. Beck, "Democratization and the 'Hidden Public.'"

36. Amy Patterson, "A Reappraisal of Democracy in Civil Society: Evidence from Rural Senegal," *Journal of Modern African Studies* 36, 3 (1998): 423–41; Nici Nelson, *African Women in the Development*

Process (London: Frank Cass, 1981); David Hirschmann, "Women and Political Participation in Africa: Broadening the Scope of Research," *World Development* 19, 12 (1991): 1679–94.

37. Human Rights Watch, "In the Shadow of Death."

38. Ibid.

39. G. Foster, C. Makufa, R. Drew, S. Kambeu, and K. Saurombe, "Supporting Children in Need through a Community-Based Orphan Visiting Programme," *AIDS Care* 8, 4 (1996): 389–403; G. Foster, R. Shakespeare, F. Chinemana, H. Jackson, S. Gregson, C. Marange, and S. Mashumba, "Orphan Prevalence and Extended Family Care in a Peri-Urban Community in Zimbabwe," *AIDS Care* 7, 1 (1995): 3–17.

40. Erick Otieno Nyambedha, Simiyu Wandibba, and Jens Aagaard-Hansen, "Policy Implications for the Inadequate Support Systems for Orphans in Western Kenya," *Health Policy* 58, 1 (2001): 83–96; UNICEF, "Children Orphaned by AIDS"; USAID, "Community Mobilization to Mitigate the Impacts of HIV/AIDS" (report on Displaced and Orphans Fund, Washington, 1999).

41. Gloria Jacques "Orphans of the AIDS Pandemic: The Sub-Saharan Africa Experience," in *AIDS and Development in Africa: A Social Science Perspective*, ed. Kempe Ronald Hope, Sr. (New York: Haworth Press, 1999), 93–108.

42. Frederick Klaits, "A Research Proposal Funded by the Social Science Research Council: Creating Parenthood and Childhood in Botswana in the Time of AIDS," *Africa Today* 44 (July–September 1999): 327–37.

43. This seems especially true if children must move to a new community, which may often be the case if their maternal grandparents care for them.

44. UNICEF, "Children Orphaned by AIDS"; Hunter and Williamson, "Children on the Brink"; White House, "Report on the Presidential Mission on Children Orphaned by AIDS in Sub-Saharan Africa: Findings and Plan of Action" (Washington: White House, 1999).

45. UNAIDS, "Children and Young People in a World of AIDS," <http://www.unaids.org/youngpeople>, 2001.

46. White House, "Presidential Mission."

47. Peter Piot, "UNAIDS Head Speaks on AIDS and Global Security," <http://usinfo.state.gov/topical/global/hiv/01100301.htm>, 2001.

48. *U.S. News and World Report*, December 18, 2000.

49. International Crisis Group, "HIV/AIDS as a Security Issue," <http://www.crisisweb.org/projects/issues/hiv_aids/reports/ A400321_19062001.pdf>, 2001.

50. *New York Times*, November 15, 1998.

51. Nelson, *African Women*.

52. G. Foster, "Orphans: Vancouver Conference Review," *AIDS Care* 9, 1 (1997): 82–87.

53. Jacques, "Orphans of the AIDS Pandemic."

54. Sidney Verba and Norman Nie, *Participation in America* (Chicago: University of Chicago Press, 1976); Tatu Vanhanen, *The Process of Democratization: A Comparative Study of 147 States, 1980–88* (New York: Crane Russak, 1990); Raymond Wolfinger and Steven Rosenstone, *Who Votes?* (New Haven: Yale University Press, 1980); Jean O'Barr, "African Women in Politics," in *African Women South of the Sahara*, ed. Margaret Hay and Sharon Stichter (New York: Longman, 1984): 140–55.

55. Alan Whiteside, quoted in *U.S. News and World Report*, December 18, 2000.

56. Human Rights Watch, "In the Shadow of Death"; Hall, *Family Coping*; UNAIDS, "Children and Young People."

57. In Kenya there are almost four million children working in the labor market, and there has been an increase in the level of prostitution, even among girls as young as nine. Human Rights Watch, "In the Shadow of Death."

58. Ibid.

59. James Segendo and Janet Nambi, "The Psychological Effect of Orphanhood: A Study of Orphans in Rakai District," *Health Transition Review: The Cultural, Social, and Behavioral Determinants of Health* 7 (suppl.) (1997): 105–24.

60. Anthony Livuza, "Malawi's AIDS Orphans Turn to Begging or Drugs," *Mail and Guardian*, July 17, 1997.

61. *Village Voice*, November 3–9, 1999.

62. Sandra Graham-Bermann and Jeffrey Edleson, eds., *Domestic Violence in the Lives of Children* (Washington, D.C.: American Psychological Association, 2001).

63. Livuza, "Malawi's AIDS Orphans"; Human Rights Watch, "In the Shadow of Death"; UNICEF, "Children Orphaned by AIDS."

64. *BBC News*, March 12, 2002.

65. Joseph, "Africa."

66. Central Intelligence Agency, "The Global Infectious Disease Threat and Its Implications for the United States," <http://www.cia. gov/cia/publications/nie/report/nie99-17d.html>, 2000.

67. Human Rights Watch, "Key Findings of the Global Report on Child Soldiers, 2001," <http://www.hrw.org/campaigns/crp/ cs-report2001.htm>, 2002.

68. Ibid; International Crisis Group, "HIV/AIDS as a Security Issue."

69. BBC News, March 12, 2002.

70. Human Rights Watch, "Getting Away with Murder, Mutilation, and Rape: New Testimony from Sierra Leone," Human Rights Watch Report 11, 3 (1999): 1.

71. Ibid.

72. USAID, "AIDS as a Developing Crisis in Africa: Rethinking Strategies and Results" (report on a consultative meeting, Washington, D.C., 1999).

73. It is certainly true that the perpetrators of the September 11 attacks on the United States were older, more educated, and more sophisticated, yet most terrorist attacks are not as well planned or well financed.

74. Cindy Combs, Terrorism in the Twenty-First Century, 2d. ed. (New York: Prentice Hall, 2000).

75. New York Times, February 13, 2002.

76. I define international donors as international organizations that are either affiliated with another country's government, such as the U.S. Agency for International Development (USAID), or that are independent from any government, such as Save the Children.

77. USAID, "Community Mobilization."

78. Hope for African Children Initiative, "Community-Based Action for Children and Families Affected by HIV/AIDS," pamphlet, Arlington, Va., n.d.

79. UNICEF, "Children Orphaned by AIDS."

80. Michael Fleshman, "AIDS Orphans: Facing Africa's 'Silent Crisis,'" Africa Recovery: Bulletin from United Nations Department of Public Information 15, 3 (2001): 1.

81. Kim Seifert, "Early Intervention: HIV/AIDS Programs for School-Aged Youth" (report for the Bureau for Africa, USAID, Washington, D.C., 1997), 5.

82. Ibid.

83. Foster, "Orphans."

84. Craig Rimmerman, *The New Citizenship* (Boulder: Westview, 1997).

85. Human Rights Watch, "In the Shadow of Death."

86. UNAIDS, "Children and Young People."

87. Louis Mwewa, "The Potential of Networks of Child-Focused Organizations," in *Orphan Alert: International Perspectives on Children Left Behind by HIV/AIDS*, formerly at <http://www.fxb.org>, n.d.

2

Civil Conflict, Sexual Violence, and HIV/AIDS

Challenges for Children in Sierra Leone

Marda Mustapha and Aiah A. Gbakima

Mary, a sixteen-year-old Sierra Leonean girl, saw both her parents killed by rebels before she was abducted. She lost her virginity when two armed rebels raped her. After she escaped, the doctors told her she needed surgery, although her family could not afford to pay.[1]

Hawa, seventeen, became pregnant after being raped. Nine months later, she gave birth to a stillborn baby. Meanwhile, Hawa was forced to become a rebel's wife. She was denied food, drugged with cocaine, and became infected with a sexually transmitted disease.[2]

Recent studies have shown that civil conflicts facilitate the spread of HIV. Matthew Smallman-Raynor and Andrew Cliff argue that civil war accounts for much of the spread of HIV in Uganda. Their argument is buttressed by regression analysis that demonstrates a strong correlation between war and disease.[3] In narrating the ordeals of refugee women who were victims of sexual violence both in war regions and refugee camps, Lynellyn Long shows how the phenomenon of sexual violence seems to be part of the pattern of civil conflicts in sub-Saharan Africa.[4] The ten-year civil war in Sierra Leone was no exception.

Throughout the ten-year rebellion by the Revolutionary United Front (RUF) in Sierra Leone, there seems to have been a systematic perpetration of sexual violence against women, girls in particular. This violence—sexual slavery, gang rape, the insertion of sticks, umbrellas, and firewood into women's vaginas[5]—was mainly the responsibility of the RUF.[6] Its victims were also exposed to severe health risks that, if not checked, could threaten the entire population of Sierra Leone, especially the children.

The Military, NGOs, and Sexual Violence

The role of civil conflicts in the spread of HIV/AIDS in sub-Saharan Africa cannot be overstated. Most determinants of the spread of HIV/AIDS in Africa—including migration (often forced), the disruption of communities, poverty, and the breakdown of law and order—are exacerbated during civil conflicts. Opportunities for sexual mixing also increase at such times, especially in refugee camps and camps for internally displaced persons (IDPs), where people of various cultural backgrounds find themselves thrown together. The result is often sexual violence, including the rape of children.

In the civil war in Sierra Leone, the military itself was the most guilty of sexual violence.[7] The military is composed of the national army, the West Side Boys, the Revolutionary United Front (RUF)/AFRC,[8] the Civil Defense Forces (CDF), and the international peacekeeping troops. Very recently, aid workers from NGOs have also been implicated as perpetrators of sexual violence. The RUF fighters were notorious for subjecting girls to gang rape. The CDF and the national army engaged in both forcible rape and statutory rape (which occurs when young girls engage in "voluntary" sex with a soldier for status, security, or food).[9] The international peacekeeping forces were mostly engaged in paying minors (below eighteen years) for sex, while aid workers traded food for sex with minors.

Rebel Forces

The rebel forces have been identified as the group most guilty of sexual violence.[10] They reportedly committed widespread gang rape and abducted young girls to be used as sex slaves. A Human Rights Watch (HRW) report notes not only widespread sexual violence but forced marriage.[11] Physicians for Human Rights (PHR) reported that the rebel forces were responsible for 93 percent of the sexual assaults during the civil conflict.[12] A documentary released by the human rights organization Witness narrates the ordeal of pretty girls, some as young as thirteen, specifically abducted by the rebel forces for sexual consumption.[13]

In February 2001, Physicians for Human Rights interviewed fifteen-year-old Bola, who was reported to be two months pregnant. She had been abducted four times since 1999:

> They held us, they cut [off] some hands, they killed some, we were taken to the bush where the sexual act was forced upon us. . . . Nine men raped me. . . . My mother was taken away. . . . I slept three days in the bush after they raped me. I was unconscious, not myself. . . . After they had raped me to their satisfaction, they left me in the bush.

This was Bola's first encounter with sexual violence through gang rape. Three others followed:

> I was taken to the base. There are many, many combatants there. There are also many other young women held there too. I was not assigned to just one man, as long as you are good looking, you have intercourse with all of them. In the third captivity, they remembered me. . . . The fourth time was last year [2000]: they did an ambush. They came for us [women], and raped us.

Bola is reported to have had two miscarriages during her unfortunate abductions. Her engagement ended when her fiancé found out about her rape. One of her miscarriages occurred after nine men raped her.[14]

Isata, also abducted by the rebels, told a similar story:

> I was a virgin before. They ruined me. . . . They undressed five of us, laid us down, used us in front of my family and took us away with them. . . . When I escaped, I couldn't walk because of the pain. I was bleeding from my vagina. . . . I can't remember how long I was held. . . . I don't want to talk because of the memories. . . . I would like to go back to school, but I can't concentrate anymore, I can't do anything.[15]

Multiple rapes became routine whenever the rebel forces captured female civilians. And sex was frequently unprotected so contracting or transmitting infections, including HIV, was likely.

Government Forces

Rape, until very recently, was not common among government forces like the CDF.[16] This situation, the HRW asserts, was because a group within the CDF, the Kamajors,[17] believed that sexual abstinence enhanced prowess in battle. However, the Kamajors were later given a greater role in national security and were deployed far from their bases. With less control by their traditional chiefs and having frequent interaction with an undisciplined Sierra Leone army, they also became increasingly undisciplined and began to practice rape—in one case a female RUF commander died of sexual torture at the hands of a senior Kamajor leader.[18]

Although none of those interviewed by PHR described sexual assaults committed by the CDF, reports existed that government forces were also involved in sexual violence against women and children during the Sierra Leone conflict. The Sierra Leone army itself was responsible for about 5 percent of the sexual assaults during the conflict.[19] These figures do not include the issue of statutory rape, which reportedly is more prevalent among the regular Sierra Leone army.

International Forces

There is no evidence that the international forces (including ECOMOG and UNAMSIL) in Sierra Leone engaged in war-related sexual violence. However, they may be guilty of statutory rape, which constitutes sexual violence, an assertion that comes from the observation that some international peace-keeping troop members target young girls for sex. While Human Rights Watch did not document any cases of rape by the Economic Community Monitoring Group (ECOMOG) or the United Nations Mission in Sierra Leone (UNAMSIL), the PHR survey shows that ECOMOG was responsible for 2 percent of the sexual assaults in the civil conflict.[20] Even though there is no hard evidence of the involvement of UNAMSIL forces in committing sexual violence, they were involved in the sexual exploitation of minors.[21] UNAMSIL soldiers were the highest bidders in the pursuit of sex with young girls, most of whom were less than eighteen years old. This bidding for sex encourages prostitution among young girls, especially those who come from impoverished families or are destitute.

The Nonmilitary Population

For a long while, no reports suggested that the nonmilitary population had engaged in sexual violence during the Sierra Leone conflict. There have, however, been some recent reports that nonmilitary populations, especially aid workers of NGOs, were involved in sexually exploiting refugees and internally displaced persons. A recent report by Save the Children found evidence, mostly through children's testimonies, that aid workers from local and international agencies—including "more than 40 aid agencies and organizations and nearly 70 individuals" in the Mano River subregion[22]—engaged in the sexual exploitation of children in exchange for food and other aid items.

So, sexual violence can take many forms. In this case, the children were not held at gunpoint, but they still found their survival threatened. Some IDPs told news organizations that "some girls said . . . it is better to love and survive than keep your pride and die of hunger." A Sierra Leonean female refugee with a two-month-old baby told an interviewer, "If you look at the need to survive during a civil war, you can conclude that a lot of girls were affected by the practice."[23]

Thus, sexual violence against women and girls is often pegged to survival on the part of the women. Aid workers control the means of survival, and it appears they use it as a tool for sexual exploitation. Men in positions of authority (both legally and illegally) take advantage of the vulnerability of women and girls. Although it also happens during peacetime, this exploitation occurs more frequently and with greater impunity during civil conflicts simply because women and girls are more vulnerable.

The Implications for HIV

Most sexual violence happened in places with few medical facilities. Most of the girls who were gang raped did not get medical attention, nor were they tested for sexually transmitted infections. The likelihood of being infected during gang rape with one or more STDs increases dramatically. And because women are biologically more vulnerable than men to such infections, the rapist, who never uses any protection, is more likely to infect the victim—especially if the rapist is HIV positive. Furthermore, the fragile reproductive systems of young girls are even more susceptible to HIV infection.[24]

The Sierra Leone army, responsible for 5 percent of sexual violence committed, has a high percentage of HIV-positive personnel. According to a report submitted to the World

Health Organization by the Associates for Global Change in 2000, of 176 soldiers and 82 civilians working for the army, 42 percent tested HIV positive. Of the 80 female soldiers that were tested, 37 percent were HIV positive.

Reports suggest that the international peacekeeping troops and aid workers seldom use condoms (this in no way suggests that the use of condoms will legitimize their actions). This scenario is troubling, because some of the soldiers serving in UNAMSIL are from countries with a very high incidence of HIV/AIDS (among them, Zambia and Kenya, whose security forces have been reported to have high rates of HIV infection).[25] Although there has been no data on the HIV rate among the UNAMSIL forces in Sierra Leone, 23 percent of 460 ECOMOG soldiers tested there in 1999 were HIV positive.[26]

Given the high rate of HIV infection in the military population in Sierra Leone, it is reasonable to assume that many of the girls who were sexually violated may have been infected with HIV. The actual number of girls who were turned into sex slaves is not known, but since most of them may not have been interviewed, or wish not to speak about it, many more of them may have been infected with HIV without their knowing.

Challenges for the Children of Sierra Leone

In 2001 the UN rated Sierra Leone the poorest country in the world and the worst country for a child to grow up in.[27] Both ratings, however, were based on economic and military statistics. There was no mention of how the war, through sexual violence, may have jeopardized the very existence of the children of Sierra Leone.

A scary implication is that Sierra Leone risks losing two generations of children. Girls face a double jeopardy: through gang rapes they may become infected with HIV or pregnant, or both. And since the virus can be transmitted from mother to child, Sierra Leone may be inheriting babies born with HIV.

The extent of children being orphaned in Sierra Leone, like the spread of HIV itself, is not known. However, given the trends of rape during civil conflict, as well as the potential for HIV infection, Sierra Leone, like other countries in sub-Saharan Africa, will likely see an upsurge in orphans through the death of infected parents. The government is ill prepared to meet such a challenge. As the pandemic grows, mortality in the general population, and among children in particular, will increase in the near future, decimating the labor force. Thus it is not far-fetched to say that the growing infection of children with HIV/AIDS will drastically impede the development of Sierra Leone.

The people of Sierra Leone, especially its children, face huge challenges ahead. With a poor health infrastructure, Sierra Leone should brace itself for a new type of war, one that, if lost, will be more devastating than the ten-year civil war that just ended. Understandably, the government has been heavily preoccupied with the rebel war, which has significantly enhanced poverty, suffering, and a range of health problems, including those posed by other illnesses, such as malaria, polio, diarrhea, and Lassa fever. Unfortunately, the HIV/AIDS pandemic was brewing and needed immediate attention. There was never the political will needed to aggressively pursue prevention nor effective health education to substantially reduce HIV transmission.

The government of Sierra Leone must now act, as only governments can, exercising the necessary political commitment to prevent further escalation of this infection among children. Administratively, the country should set up a national HIV/AIDS task force to develop a national policy and secure the resources needed to address the pandemic.[28] A commitment of political will at the highest level in Sierra Leone is needed. The effectiveness of such political will has been demonstrated elsewhere, especially in Uganda and Senegal.[29]

A national AIDS task force would be able to embark on an education campaign that focuses on educating children about their rights and the dangers of having early or unprotected sex. Children can become aware of their rights through counseling, both in schools and other community centers.[30] Zimbabwe has been doing this for the past ten years and it has helped slow down infection rates among teenagers. Educating children about their human rights, safe sex, and abstinence is especially effective when the government protects their legal rights as well.[31] For example, the age of sexual consent could be increased from sixteen to eighteen. In addition, HIV-infected children should be monitored, ensuring they have access to health care.

Notes

For their critical comments, we thank Carol Thompson, Mary Ann Steger, and the graduate students in the Political Science Department of Northern Arizona University, especially Kurt Fenske.

1. Physicians for Human Rights, *War-Related Sexual Violence in Sierra Leone: A Population-Based Assessment* (Boston: Physicians for Human Rights, 2002), 73.

2. Ibid., 68.

3. Matthew Smallman-Raynor and Andrew Cliff, "Civil War and the Spread of AIDS in Central Africa," *Epidemiological Infections*, 1991, 69–80, 107.

4. Lynellyn Long, "Refugee Women, Violence, and HIV," in *Sexual Cultures and Migration in the Era of AIDS*, ed. Gilbert Herdt (Oxford: Clarendon Press, 1996).

5. Human Rights Watch, *World Report 2001: Sierra Leone*, <www.hrw.org/backgrounder/africa/sl-bck0226.htm>.

6. Physicians for Human Rights, *Sexual Violence*, 51–53.

7. For a definition of military population, see Rodger Yeager and S. J. Kingma, "AIDS Brief: Military Populations" (USAID/WHO, 2000).

8. Below we will refer to the RUF/AFRC as the rebel forces.

9. We consider it sexual violence when an adult fighter engages in any sexual activity with a minor. Army officers in Sierra Leone always had a ready supply of food since they were supplied with bags of rice, the country's staple food.

10. Physicians for Human Rights, *Sexual Violence*, 44, 51–53.

11. Human Rights Watch, *World Report*.

12. Physicians for Human Rights, *Sexual Violence*, 44.

13. Lilibet Foster, *Operation Fine Girl: Rape Used as a Weapon of War in Sierra Leone* (New York: Witness, 2001), videocassette.

14. Interview, Port Loko, Sierra Leone, in Physicians for Human Rights, *Sexual Violence*, 64–70.

15. Interview, Freetown, Sierra Leone, in Physicians for Human Rights, *Sexual Violence*, 69–70.

16. Human Rights Watch, *World Report*.

17. The Kamajors are traditional warriors from the Mende ethnic group in Sierra Leone.

18. Human Rights Watch, *World Report*.

19. Physicians for Human Rights, *Sexual Violence*, 49.

20. Ibid.

21. The last word in the streets of Freetown, Sierra Leone's capital, is "the UNAMSIL dollar factor." Young men lament that UNAMSIL soldiers exploit young girls by paying for sex with dollars.

22. *United Nations High Commissioner for Refugees and Save the Children Report, 2002.* The Mano River subregion includes Sierra Leone, Guinea, and Liberia.

23. Associated Press, February 2002.

24. UNAIDS, *AIDS Epidemic Update: December 2000* (Geneva: UNAIDS, 2000).

25. World Health Organization, *Country Reports for Zambia and Kenya*, (Geneva, 2000).

26. Associates for Global Change; WHO, "HIV/AIDS in Sierra Leone: The Future at Stake" (report by Associates for Global Change, December 2000).

27. *U.N. Development Report 2001* (New York: United Nations).

28. World Bank, *Confronting AIDS: Public Priorities in a Global Epidemic* (Washington, D.C.: World Bank, 1997).

29. UNICEF, *Children Orphaned by AIDS: Frontline Responses from Eastern and Southern Africa* (New York: UNICEF, 1999), 7.

30. Ibid.

31. Ibid.

3

The Vulnerability of Children and Orphaned Youth in Zimbabwe

Prisca N. Nemapare and D. Dow Tang

Terminal illness and death are traumatic—whether a parent loses a child or a child loses a parent. The loss of a father, the symbol of financial security, results in untold worry about the future. Not having a mother, who will love, nurture, and guide you, is one of the most difficult things for any child to handle. Such suffering among children has been one of the consequences of the HIV/AIDS pandemic.[1]

Current official HIV/AIDS statistics for Zimbabwe are grim at best.[2] AIDS has devastated the country for many years now and shows no signs of subsiding. Nationally, two thousand deaths occur each week (some say it's more like thirty-five hundred). Those with AIDS occupy 80 percent of all hospital beds. Among the most affected age group, fifteen- to thirty-nine-year-olds, 66 percent are HIV positive. Among the very young (under five), AIDS causes 75 percent of all pediatric deaths. It is also estimated that 38 percent of all pregnant women in the metropolitan areas are HIV positive. The population growth rate of Zimbabwe is declining; it was 3.1 percent in 2002 as compared to 3.6 percent in 1980.

In 1999 it was estimated that there were nine hundred thousand AIDS orphans in Zimbabwe.[3] By 2002 the HIV/AIDS pandemic was generating six hundred thousand orphans annually. The burden of caring for these children is born by women (grandmothers and widows), and for grandmothers this responsibility continues almost to the grave.

In such a scenario children and the elderly are among the most vulnerable to poverty. In Zimbabwe poverty is much more pronounced in rural areas, where 70 percent of the population still resides. It is estimated that 86 percent of the nation's population is living below the poverty line.[4] Women and children, constituting the majority of people who live in poverty, are the most vulnerable to HIV/AIDS. This is especially true among the young because of dependent status within the family.

In 1999 an ongoing survey began on AIDS orphans in Masvingo and Matabeleland South Provinces. Interviews with more than 1,510 children revealed that they have aged caregivers, are at risk of abandonment, suffer threats to their health and nutrition, and lack security, basic rights, sufficient community support, and a proper nurturing environment.

Children as Heads of Households

As a result of the loss of one or more parents, some children are now heads of households—without any experience, education, or resources. They are raising their younger siblings—a daunting responsibility even for adults. These children are uncertain how to move forward with their lives and wonder how they will cope with what has happened to them. Such children have lost all childhood characteristics because they have had to grow up quickly after being orphaned. Undertaking such roles, with little or no resources, has resulted in some becoming involved in behaviors that are detrimental to their well-being.

Children's Rights

Some orphaned children are left with one parent or are taken in by a relative. These children are expected to carry out a variety of chores around the home. Such tasks are normal; however, some of the tasks are heavy and interfere with schooling. Reading, telling stories, and simply playing are abandoned. Often, instead of going to school, children are sent to the gristmill, located at a distance, to have maize ground into flour. Sometimes a stepmother or guardian keeps an orphaned ward at home doing chores, while allowing their own children to go to school. Feeling that no one cares is overwhelming for a child in such circumstances and may lead to depression, bad behavior, or difficulty in coping with life—and eventually perhaps to crime, promiscuity, or running away from home.

Elderly Care Providers and Community Support

A majority (52 percent) of caregivers in the survey are grandparents, who because of their age have little energy, resources, or physical capacity to deal with young children. Grandparents had the largest number of children (822) in their care (six per individual). Widowed mothers had the next largest number of children (408), followed by siblings (76), widowed fathers (56), and other relatives (28). Widows and widowers, as well as other older relatives involved in the care of orphans, all require extra moral support for such a demanding job.

In a traditional and cultural sense, child rearing is a community effort. Most orphaned children, as well as the care providers, had no one to talk to or confide in. After a while, pent-up emotions are liable to burst—the consequences of which can be disastrous for both children and caregivers. In the current study, grandparents (grandmothers, in particular) cared for too many orphaned children. Teachers, neighbors, and community members and their leaders should form a community support system aimed at assisting such households. Most grandparents have never been to school, and others have schooling only up to the fourth grade. Low levels of education render them virtually incapable of helping children with schoolwork, let alone appreciating the importance of a good education. The community support network should be responsible for providing educators who can meet the special needs of orphaned children and youth. Without this support, the children and their caregivers are being condemned to a life of poverty and a bleak future.

Abandonment and the Loss of Security

In Zimbabwe the father symbolizes personal and financial security. His death means the loss of this safety. The death of both parents is even more difficult for a child. Children get angry at the world because one or both parents have died. When this happens, they have no one to talk to—no one who can explain to them what has happened and why. Counseling is needed to allow these children to accept what has happened and forge ahead with their lives.

Some men and women abandon their children once a spouse dies of HIV/AIDS. Neither the children nor the grandparents know the whereabouts of the parent. Abandoned children feel worthless and end up blaming themselves. The resulting bad behavior patterns may include poor attendance at school, dropping out of school altogether, and property destruction.

In the traditional culture, children are punished when they do something wrong; however, the parent or guardian usually explains why such action has been taken. This is not the case with a majority of orphans. Sometimes punishment may include being deprived of supper for several days. Such punishment is detrimental to the nutritional and emotional well-being of the child and, ultimately, to his or her physical health.

A Nurturing Environment and Behavior

For some of the children in the survey, teachers and care providers reported behavioral problems that included being bullied or bullying others, getting into fights, and stealing. Such behaviors call for a cohesive community support system that shows zero tolerance of children being abusive to others and zero tolerance for child abuse by adults.

An unsupportive home environment is hardest on teenagers because adolescence is in itself a difficult stage of life. Being an orphan during the teen years can be extremely depressing. A positive, safe, and caring home environment is the cornerstone of the child's future, providing impetus for proper growth, development, and preparation to be a productive member of society. It is essential for caregivers and the orphaned children to have a solid community support system.

Individuals who form part of this support system must be worthy of respect, compassionate, reliable, strong, and uncompromising in character. It would not be useful to select individuals who may feel overwhelmed by the responsibility, as they might later prove unreliable.

For children who were born and grew up in an urban environment prior to being orphaned, being absorbed into a surrogate rural family can be a traumatic experience. There is little privacy in rural areas. This can cause a difficult adjustment.

The cousins they may be living with may be complete strangers to them. Suddenly these orphans find themselves having to share blankets and clothes and doing chores they may never have done before. They may have to change schools and may have to walk a long distance to get there. Others have to make new friends or learn new languages. Such living conditions add to the physical and psychological burden orphans are already carrying.

In spite of all the difficulties that orphans may be living under, some show a high degree of hope. Orphans in the present study were aware that they needed to remain in school. They firmly believed that with an education their circumstances would change for the better. They described aspirations that must be encouraged and cultivated. They dreamt of becoming teachers, nurses, law enforcement officers, soldiers, nuns, doctors, drivers, engineers, secretaries.

Health and Nutrition

Personal hygiene, proper sanitation, and access to clean water were some of the biggest health issues faced by the families in the study. Interviews with orphans and caregivers revealed that well over 50 percent of the households surveyed had no toilets and many lacked clean water and stable access to food and the money for school fees. Caregivers complained bitterly about the distance to the health center and the cost for health care, which made it difficult to receive information and to get health care to children who needed it.

The average caregiver's household had between five and six children, and they came from three or four previous families in which at least one parent had died. Typically, a grandmother who has only a hut for sleeping and another for cooking takes in all these children. In such congested living arrangements, with inadequate ventilation and space, communicable diseases, fungal infections, intestinal parasites, and diarrhea become rampant. Coupled with inadequate nutrition, the situation can easily deteriorate, resulting in multiple epidemics.

In 2001, 70 percent of the households harvested fewer than five bags of maize, and that figure rose to nearly 90 percent in 2002, which was officially declared a drought year in Zimbabwe. Since this low production means less food and less money for clothing and school fees, such conditions, experienced for an extended period, will be detrimental to both health and school performance.

As the educational level of caregivers is low and poverty is quite high, it is therefore unlikely children will receive adequate daily nutrition. In 2001 both the quality and quantity of nutrients needed by growing children fell well below requirements set by the UN World Health Organization.[5]

With such large numbers of children being malnourished and not being properly educated, the future development of Zimbabwe is grossly compromised. Many AIDS orphans are not in school because of a lack of money or because they are responsible for younger siblings or sick parents. Those in school may not perform well as a result of poor nutrition and health, depression, and worry about their current circumstances and the future. Such a situation presents a serious crisis with respect to child survival in Zimbabwe.

Notes

1. United Nations Children's Fund, *The Progress of Nations* (New York: UNICEF, 2000); Zimbabwe, *Poverty in Zimbabwe* (Harare: Central Statistical Office, 1998).

2. UNDP, "Poverty Reduction Forum, and AIDS 1998," in Brian Raftopoulos, Tony Hawkins, and Dede-Esi Amanor-Wilks, *Zimbabwe Human Development Report, 1998* (Harare: UNDP, 1998); Zimbabwe, *Zimbabwe National Report* (Harare: Central Statistical Office, 1992).

3. UNAIDS, United Nations, New York, 2000; World Health Organization, *The World Health Report* (Geneva: WHO, 2000).

4. World Bank, *Intensifying Action against HIV/AIDS in Africa: Responding to Development Crisis* (Washington, D.C.: World Bank, 2000).

5. United Nations, Administrative Committee on Coordination, Subcommittee on Nutrition, *Fourth Report on the World Nutrition Situation: Nutrition throughout the Life Cycle* (Geneva: United Nations, 2000).

4

Reducing the Vulnerability of Africa's Children to HIV/AIDS

Michael J. Kelly

Kelvin had been in good steady employment as a cook, but he had to stop work because of increasing sickness and depression. He was the father of five children. The first died from malaria, when only an infant. The second survived. The third was found dead, having fallen into an empty swimming pool at the house where Kelvin worked. The fourth had HIV, transmitted from her mother, and died before her third birthday. The fifth child, who was born a few days before Kelvin himself died of AIDS, lived for only a few weeks. Kelvin's wife, the mother of the five children, herself died of AIDS less than two years after Kelvin. Nobody had survived from the family except the second-born, Bwalya.

Kelvin's older brother, Rogers, made room in his small home and among his own four children for Bwalya, by now about nine years old. But Rogers was also infected with HIV. For six months he alternated between living at home and living in a hospital. As he wasted away, he experienced much nausea and could no longer take the drugs for the tuberculosis that was ravaging his lungs. Eventually he died in the hospital, dreadfully emaciated, but peacefully and with dignity.

Miyanda, the widow of Rogers, worked hard to care for her own children, ranging in age from one to nine years. She also kept Bwalya in the family, since he had no other living relatives that anybody knew about. Miyanda managed to get employment as a cleaner and out of her small income ensured that Bwalya and her older children attended school. But within a year she began to have periodic bouts of weakness and illness. Diagnosed as having tuberculosis, at first she responded well to the treatment but later began to lose weight at an alarming rate. Less than eighteen months after the death of her husband, Rogers, she too was close to death. The wife of a male relative moved into her house to look after her and the children. But all who knew her believed that little could be done for her and that she would survive for no more than a few days.

At this stage, Miyanda's employer made a generous decision. Agreeing with his family that he could just about afford the cost of treatment ($75 a month), he brought Miyanda to a clinic for AIDS patients and asked for her to be put on antiretroviral therapy. The treatment was started, and Miyanda survived her crisis. Within three weeks she was back home, still weak and thin, but alive and getting stronger every day. Two months later she was well enough to be able to resume employment and undertake some light cleaning duties. That is how her condition remains at present. Without the therapy she would be dead. But with the drugs she is alive and able to work, and her children are not orphaned.

Meanwhile, Bwalya has continued to attend school. As he enters adolescence, he is rather reserved. He knows that he is on his own. He has lost not only father and mother but all his siblings. In his new home he underwent yet again the experience of being orphaned when his uncle died. The world that was building up for him came perilously close to falling apart when his uncle's wife was near to death. If she had died, Bwalya would have had nobody left in the world except his cousins, all younger than himself. A deep sadness attaches to him; laughter does not seem to be part of his life. He plays with his cousins, but halfheartedly. Life has hurt him very deeply. He could scarcely bear it if it hurt him again.

The Reality of Childhood

The World Summit for Children has affirmed that childhood should be a time of joy and peace, of playing, learning, and growing.[1] But for Bwalya, as for millions of the children of Africa, the reality of childhood has been altogether different. Coping repeatedly with death, grief, and mourning, without mother or father to give care and loving attention, moving from one home to another, not knowing how long the present situation might last, Bwalya's childhood has been anything but laughter-filled, innocent, and happy. His experiences have aged him before his time, transforming him into a "juvenile adult"—vulnerable, scarred, and wary of life.

Yet Bwalya has been more fortunate than many others. He still has a home, a family to which he belongs, and an aunt who takes care of him as she takes care of her own children. For millions of children in Africa the reality of childhood is much more harsh. The turmoil of war and conflict; spartan living conditions within refugee settlements; the endless daily struggle for enough food to tide them over to the next day's struggle; sickness, weariness, and lack of physical comfort; the absence of psychological and emotional support; sexual and economic exploitation; and the experience of violence and abuse have all denied these children their time of playing, laughter, and learning.

Bwalya's experience shows that HIV/AIDS is leading to a vast number of orphans. Almost every strategy for responding to this challenge starts from the assumption that there will be enormous growth in the number of children who will be orphaned by HIV/AIDS, and each strategy tries to devise ways of ensuring their satisfactory human survival. One could ask, however, for more attention to forestalling the challenge and for greater concern about broad strategies for stemming the suffering of children whose mothers are infected with HIV.

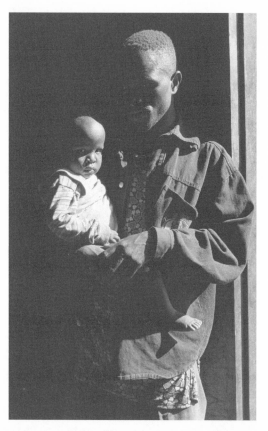

Fig. 4.1. At the doorway of their tin hut in Zambia, a young HIV-positive father holds his young HIV-positive son. The man's wife died of AIDS, a fate that awaits both the father and the son. Photograph by Andrew Petkun. Used with permission.

Responding to the Needs of
Children of HIV-Infected Mothers

There are two issues here: keeping mothers alive and healthy, and keeping their children alive and healthy. Arguably, a child's greatest need is for a healthy mother who can provide the care, support, and nurturing that will see the child through her years of childhood. Without the mother the family may fall apart. If she is infected with a life-threatening condition, everything possible should be done to keep her alive. Not only does the mother have a personal fundamental right to live, she is also essential to preventing the disintegration of families.

Family disintegration, and the concomitant increase in the number of orphans, can be stemmed by making antiretroviral treatment available for every HIV-positive mother who has young children. Treatment will allow mothers to raise their children in a nurturing environment. Thailand has already embarked on such a program.[2] The countries of Africa should be enabled to do the same.

The life-long provision of antiretroviral therapy for these mothers will be at significant economic cost. But it is a cost that will preclude even more costly economic and social outlays if orphan numbers continue to rise and families fall apart. In addition to the human suffering, trauma, and grief that orphans experience, the growth in their number is leading in many countries to situations where unanticipated educational, social, economic, and security problems are undermining existing systems and coping mechanisms. These problems can be forestalled by keeping mothers alive so that the number of orphans does not grow.

Keeping children alive in the midst of the HIV/AIDS epidemic entails therapy to reduce parent-to-child transmission of HIV; antiretroviral therapy for those children who, in spite of such treatment, remain HIV positive; and antiretroviral

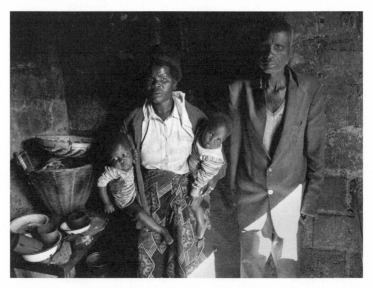

Fig. 4.2. A forty-two-year-old Zambian woman standing beside her eighty-one-year-old husband holds her two-year-old son in one arm and her two-year-old HIV-positive grandson in the other. Photograph by Andrew Petkun. Used with permission.

therapy for all children who contract HIV in their childhood years. No child should ever be required to carry the burden of HIV, let alone AIDS. Perhaps the Convention on the Rights of the Child should be amended to include the right of every child to freedom from HIV/AIDS.

Sexually Transmitted HIV among Children

Because of the low nutritional status of women, the poverty of families, and the inadequacy of medical services, many children in Africa die in their first two or three years. Few of those born to HIV-positive mothers receive the medical care, attention, nutrients, and stimulation that would enable them to live for ten or more years. In the absence of interventions, the likelihood is that 30 percent or more of them will be infected with HIV. The majority of these children will die in their first five years.

Treatment with the AIDS drug nevirapine, which is readily available, relatively inexpensive, and easily administered, can greatly reduce the possibility of mother-to-child transmission of HIV. Currently in Africa, one can expect that even when nevirapine is administered 10 percent or more of the infants born to seropositive mothers will themselves continue to be seropositive and will remain so until, after a few brief years of suffering, they succumb to an AIDS-related opportunistic infection.

But these are not the only young children infected with HIV. Many become infected through sexual abuse, all too frequently within their own family circle. Pedophilia appears to know no national or cultural boundaries. Neither does incest. The occurrence of the two has proved a lethal combination for many children, leading to severe psychosocial trauma and in some cases to the transmission of HIV.

Sexual Abuse in the Home

The parents of a three-year-old girl were deeply disturbed at attempts by the child to have oral sex with her father. Investigations revealed the origins of the problem. The mother's brother had initiated the child into the practice. Children are highly vulnerable to sexual exploitation.

An ancient myth that having sexual intercourse with a virgin could cure certain diseases has reemerged in Africa, the Caribbean, and other parts of the world in two chilling forms. The desire to have sex with a virgin leads to sexual exploitation and rape of young girls, including babies. This sexual exploitation results in physical and emotional damage and often the HIV infection of young girls. The other manifestation of this myth is that having sex with a young person with physical or mental handicap will cure AIDS, leading to the sexual exploitation and risk of HIV infection of highly vulnerable boys and girls who are incapable of defending themselves. Both of these aberrant practices probably derive from the self-justification of adults who, fearing that an adult partner may be HIV positive, turn to those who are presumed to be HIV free. Subsequently they seek to excuse their actions by maintaining that they were seeking an AIDS cure.

HIV-infected Schoolchildren

The pattern of AIDS cases in Zambia is typical of what has been reported from countries and regions elsewhere (fig. 4.3). AIDS cases fall off significantly between ages five and fourteen, but from age fifteen onward, they grow rapidly, with no evidence of decline until the mid-thirties or early forties. AIDS cases among those between fifteen and nineteen show a marked increase over the number of such cases among those between five and fourteen; the increase for young women is particularly noteworthy.

The above numbers deal with AIDS cases, not HIV infection. Progression from initial HIV infection to clinical AIDS

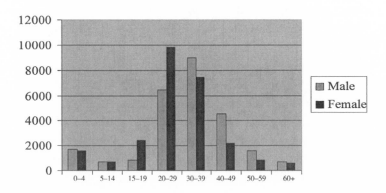

Fig 4.3. Cumulative AIDS Cases by Age and Gender, Zambia

symptoms occurs slowly, over several years. In Africa, the high background level of infections other than HIV, the presence of a variety of debilitating parasites (especially malarial), and the generally low nutritional status of much of the population may contribute to a more rapid progression of the disease. Nevertheless, even in Africa one can expect a period of five years or more to elapse between initial HIV infection and the development of AIDS.[3]

Boys and girls who show symptoms of AIDS between the ages of fifteen and nineteen must have become infected with HIV at much younger ages. Preteen and early-teen infections are realities that deserve much greater attention than they receive. Unfortunately, existing methods do not capture information on the frequency of such infections, though anecdotal information exists. Thus, on the assumption that an average of seven years elapses between HIV infection and eventual death from AIDS, death records for the Eastern Cape, South Africa, imply that almost 5 percent of a sample of 1,424 AIDS cases acquired HIV before their fifteenth birthday.[4]

In the absence of good information, young people below the age of fifteen tend to be classified into a uniform HIV-free "window of hope." They are seen as constituting a special audience to whom prevention messages should be targeted. However, if any among these young persons should be HIV positive, few of the messages will speak to them about the value of a healthy lifestyle in prolonging or improving the quality of their lives. They will be considered too young to be encouraged to have themselves counseled and tested, and in any case it is unlikely that at present adequate testing services would be available or that those available would be "friendly" to youngsters aged fourteen or younger. This situation needs to be addressed so that these children can be tested, counseled, and receive medical support.

School as a Site for Potential HIV Infection

Preteen and teenage HIV infection occurs mainly through sexual activity. Demographic health surveys show that about one-third of young women and one-half of young men in Zambia become sexually experienced by their mid-teens. This sexual activity occurs among young people themselves and between young people and adults. In both cases it may carry the risk of HIV transmission and infection. In Africa, a number of school-related circumstances heighten these risks.

First, there is considerable age mixing in classes at school, particularly in rural schools. Age mixing leads to sex between older boys and younger girls, which has a high risk for HIV transmission. The risk for the younger girl is that the older boy, having been exposed to more sex partners, may be HIV positive.[5]

Schoolchildren rarely calculate the HIV risk underlying their sexual activity. Nevertheless, because of factors that delay a child's entry to school (such as the distance between home and school and the costs associated with schooling) and factors that prolong the duration of schooling (such as the stop-start pattern displayed by many rural children, whose families depend on the periodic labor they can provide), the same class may contain students whose ages range from seven to sixteen, or whose sexual development ranges from the naïve and ignorant to the knowledgeable and experienced. This heightens the risk of sexual activity, often playing a key role in the transmission of HIV infection.

A Wide Range of Ages within a Class

- In a school where the defined age range for seventh grade is thirteen to fourteen, one boy confessed that he was nineteen years old.

- Enumerators gathering data for national censuses have encountered boys and girls who are seven and more years older than the regulation age for the school grade to which they say they belong.
- In a large survey of fifth grade pupils (who should be about twelve years old), fewer than a quarter were of the correct age. Almost one-third were less than twelve, another third were thirteen to fourteen, and about one-seventh were from fifteen to eighteen. On average, boys were eight months older than girls.[6]

Another contributing risk factor is the long distance between the homes of many rural children and the school they attend, a distance that many traverse daily by a set route on foot. The risks of sexual harassment, from older pupils or from adults encountered on the way to or from school, deter a number of African parents from sending their girls to school once they reach puberty.

Boarding schools and school hostels are a time-honored response to the problems of distance and scattered populations. Single-sex boarding schools increase opportunities for homosexual activity among students. Opportunities for heterosexual sex with residents from the surrounding area or with students of a nearby school also increase.

Countries in Africa that are grappling with ways of expanding secondary school coverage for very scattered rural populations now recognize the HIV/AIDS implications of their decisions. Mozambique, where development has long been held back by colonialism and civil war, is proceeding cautiously in its efforts to increase the number of secondary school students. Policymakers weigh the relative merits of large boarding schools that can offer a rich and varied curriculum but carry attendant risks for HIV transmission against smaller day schools, located within communities, where the potential for HIV transmission would be less.[7]

School as a Locus for Coerced Sex and Rape

In addition to seeking sexual encounters, many young people have sex thrust upon them. Relatively speaking, in Africa higher proportions of young people, especially girls, may be initiated into sex by older men than by their peers. Much of the sex experienced by young girls is either rape or sex elicited through moral, economic, or academic pressure. Moral pressure is applied when the girl fears the ending of an emotionally valued relationship; economic pressure takes the form of the girl having to forego the material remunerations that come with sexual compliance; and academic pressure takes the form of sex with a teacher that may lead to advancement in school, the award of higher grades, or a preview of examination questions.

School-Related Violence and Sexual Abuse in South Africa

- South African girls continue to be raped, sexually abused, sexually harassed, and assaulted at school by male classmates and teachers. For many South African girls, violence and abuse are an inevitable part of the school environment.[8]
- Thirty-three percent of South African women raped before age fifteen were attacked by teachers, another 21 percent by relatives, and a similar number by strangers or acquaintances.[9]

While young schoolgirls are humiliated and sexually violated in this way, their parents often believe schools protect their children, contributing to their preparation for a responsible adult sexual life. Yet the harsh reality, which parents, education authorities, and the public at large do not take sufficiently into account, is that the school may constitute a high-risk situation for many young people, especially girls. It may be a focal area for sexual harassment and rape, with considerable potential for HIV transmission.

Malnutrition and the Risk of HIV Infection

Hunger, undernourishment, and poorly balanced diets are the lot of millions in Africa. Poverty afflicts broad swaths of a continent where some 220 million people live on less than a dollar a day.[10] These numbers translate into tens of millions of suffering children. While their life should be one of joy, learning, and health it is one of grief, anxiety, and malnutrition.

When testing her students' ability to understand oral questions, a Zambian teacher asked one twelve-year-old girl, "What kind of food did you eat yesterday?" At first, the embarrassed child muttered something unintelligible. Then, under repeated questioning and coaxing, she said, "I did not eat yesterday because it was not my turn to eat, but I will eat today." While the girl's reply shocked the teacher, it drew little reaction from the rest of the class. Undoubtedly children all over Africa have had similar experiences.

Currently, a clearer understanding is emerging of the implications of malnutrition for HIV transmission and for the infection's accelerated progression to AIDS. A strong correlation exists between HIV prevalence on the one hand and the inadequate protein and calorie consumption of Africa's children on the other.[11] As the media pictures of children with scabious skin and inflamed eyes show, malnutrition weakens the skin and mucous membranes. Instead of being the first line of defense against infection during a sexual encounter, the thin, torn, ulcerated skin and mucous membranes in a malnourished child's genital areas provide ready entry for viral infections of all kinds, including HIV.

By the same token, HIV/AIDS contributes to malnutrition. HIV and AIDS have a negative impact on household economies—through reduction in income, a decline in productive capacity, and a wide range of AIDS-related expenses.[12] Household food security is impaired because of reductions both in production and in the resources available to purchase food. In households in which an adult has AIDS less time is dedicated to child care, hygiene, and food preparation. Food consumption generally decreases, while malnutrition becomes salient.[13] The result is an increase in the classic signs of malnutrition—stunting, underweight, wasting—among children. Some 56 percent of young children (under five years of age) in Zambia currently show clinical signs of malnutrition, compared with 46 percent five years ago. HIV/AIDS has clearly abetted this increase.

Households Headed by Children

The AIDS pandemic is also directly responsible for the emergence of a relatively new sociological phenomenon—the household in which there is no adult member, and where, by unspoken consent, usually the oldest child assumes economic and quasi-parenting responsibility for siblings. Children who head households of this nature may be from ten to twelve years old or more. Communities usually intervene when all those in the household are prepubescent. Bwalya lost both his parents and his uncle to AIDS (as noted above), and it was only because his aunt was kept alive that he did not have to take responsibility for his four younger cousins.

The peak ages for AIDS deaths in Africa are twenty-five to thirty-five for females and thirty-five to forty-five for males. AIDS is claiming the lives of a high proportion of young mothers and fathers when their children are still young. On the death of the parents, efforts may be made to entrust the orphaned children to the care of other relatives. However, various problems may interfere. There may be no surviving close relatives who can absorb the orphans into their households, or the households of surviving relatives may have reached their absorptive capacity. For example, all the brothers and sisters of a senior government official in southern Africa have succumbed to AIDS, leaving him with the financial and parenting responsibility for more than fifty nephews and nieces.

The issue of location can also arise when placing the orphaned children in the home of a relative. If the children were reared in an urban area and their only surviving relatives live far away in the countryside, clashing cultures, rootlessness, and language differences may make it difficult for the rural family to integrate the urban children, and for the urban children to adapt to the rural situation.

The close ties developed between siblings during their early childhood and especially during the traumatic final months before the death of their parents often bind them very closely together. A guiding principle in programming for orphan support is that, as far as possible, sibling groups should not be dismantled. Siblings depend very extensively on one another for support, comfort, and a sense of belonging; they feel highly vulnerable when apart. In many cases, as AIDS progressively wastes their parents, they quietly assume responsibility for the household, including care of their parents, and of their own affairs. Cemented into unity by their common trauma and suffering, they are reluctant to let go of that solidarity after their parents' deaths. Being with one another brings meaning and a sense of belonging into their shattered young lives.

Adults find it hard to appreciate the challenges confronting the members of a child-headed household. Alice's problems, discussed below, may be extreme but are not altogether unusual. Most child-headed households experience a never-ending struggle to get the basic necessities of life: food, clean water, fuel, shelter, clothing, basic medicines, and education. The child heading the household may be in charge, directing the operations of the others, but the participation of all members is needed to ensure that they eat, are clothed, and have a place they can call home. Almost certainly, household responsibilities will mean that the oldest can no longer attend school. The attendance of others will depend greatly on the resourcefulness of the one heading the household and on the vision of a better future that schooling may hold—something that differs from country to country. But because the first priority is survival, many of those in child-headed households look for ways to obtain food and income. This quest drives many children onto the streets, swelling the number of street children. It leads some into petty theft. It induces young girls into the sale of sex. It drives all of them downward into a further spiral of poverty and risk of HIV infection.

Alice, a Child Mother

Alice, a thirteen-year-old girl with responsibility for three younger brothers and sisters, had been heading her household since she was eleven. She was twelve when she became pregnant. Because taking care of her AIDS-afflicted mother had been her preoccupation for several years, Alice never learned how to care for an infant. She delivered her baby alone at home and after cleaning herself walked over to the neighbor's home to ask how she should bathe the baby and take care of it.

Models of Care for Orphans and Vulnerable Children

Child-headed households represent one extreme on the continuum of caring for AIDS orphans. Other solutions exist:

- relocation of orphaned siblings into the households of relatives;
- repatriation of orphans to the village from which one of the parents originally came;
- maintenance of orphans in the original home, but as an adjunct to an adult-headed household that monitors, supervises, guides, and assumes some responsibility;
- maintenance of the orphans' sibling group, but with the protection, support, and basic household skills coming

through relatively informal community-based day care centers;

- foster home arrangements for individual orphans;
- arranging for the adoption of orphans;
- temporary placement of orphans in a transit home while more permanent arrangements are being made;
- placement of orphaned children in an orphanage.

Most solutions recognize that the primary response to the challenge of the growing number of orphans must come from families and communities. The least satisfactory response is institutional placement, not merely because of the cost but, more important, because the place for a child is in a family, not in an institutionalized setting. However, sometimes placement in an orphanage may be in the best interests of the child.

Community-Managed Day Care Centers for Orphans

The Kenneth Kaunda Children of Africa Foundation has established day care centers in five high-density locations in Lusaka, Zambia, each catering to twenty or more orphans between three and nine years old. The orphans continue to live with their grandparents (or other elderly family members) but attend one of the centers during the day. Here they get meals and basic education. They also receive medical treatment at an AIDS clinic run by the foundation. The clinic has noted that the regular, nutritious diet it provides has protected many of the children from needing medical attention, even those who are HIV-infected. Widows from neighboring communities are responsible for the day-to-day running of the centers.

Many compelling questions about the welfare of AIDS orphans still remain to be answered:

- If children are placed with elderly relatives—the only surviving kinfolk in a society that is severely affected by AIDS—who will care for these elderly caregivers?

- What provisions can be made for the transmission of social, household, agricultural, cultural, and other skills to children, when a large proportion of those possessing such skills have already died?[14]
- How can one ensure that a family that takes responsibility for an orphan will provide for the child's basic needs for love, food, health care, and education on an equal footing with the children born in the household?
- What assistance can be given to enable children whose parents have died of AIDS to cope with their loss and to deal with the trauma of observing their parents die?
- What steps can be taken to transform cultural perspectives that do not encourage deep, personal manifestations of grief, especially on the part of boys?
- How will today's orphans become tomorrow's parents when they will never have known the formative years of a normal childhood, being parented in a normal family with father, mother, brothers, and sisters?
- Will the increase in the number of orphaned juveniles as a proportion of the general population lead to an increase in crime levels in the short to medium term?[15]

A New Vision of Schooling

Questions also arise about formal schooling. From several perspectives, school attendance emerges as one of the best antidotes for the problems that confront an HIV/AIDS orphan. A school epitomizes normality, and normality may be what orphans and vulnerable children need more than anything else. Schools can provide stability in the face of parental death, social relocation, and the accompanying uncertainty. Schools also symbolize a hope for the future. With much of their past buried with their parents, orphans need the help that schools can provide in orienting them toward the future.

But conventional schooling tends to be inflexible in terms of daily schedules, calendars, and methods of delivery. It is also, almost by definition, tied to a physical location. This arrangement hinders the participation of orphans, especially those who head households. Moreover, while the theory underlying the school curriculum generally allows for considerable diversity and adaptation in response to local and learner needs, its practice may be very different. Teachers are often obliged to cover a set content (sometimes with a view to examination requirements) in a specified time. This curriculum straitjacket constrains all but the most creative teachers from responding imaginatively to the perceived needs of orphans and vulnerable children. It also inhibits the school from introducing or emphasizing the teaching and learning of practical skills that may be of prime importance to most of its children. The question, then, is how to free up the conventional school system so that it can respond more flexibly and imaginatively to the real needs of all children, especially orphans. The various paradigms of educational provision have never proved fully satisfactory, even in an AIDS-free world. Something new and completely different has long been needed and is needed even more urgently now because of the challenges presented by HIV/AIDS. The new schooling models would likely be deeply rooted in the community, with broader grassroots participation, responsibility, and authority.

A cardinal principle for a country affected by HIV/AIDS should be to reduce the vulnerability of its children to HIV infection. There are three reasons for this:

- Children have equal rights with other members of the human family.

- Children are most vulnerable—physically, mentally, socially, and economically—to HIV/AIDS and its consequences.
- A country's future depends on the well-being of its children.

To address the vulnerability of children necessitates the prevention of further growth of the AIDS epidemic and management of its present impacts. Maintaining the existence of the family, which is the natural environment for the growth and well-being of children, is an essential way of keeping children from becoming orphaned. The principal need is for strategies that will keep families alive and strengthen their capacities to care for their children. In practical terms, this calls for interventions to keep both parents, especially mothers, alive; strengthening health services; strengthening educational provision; and strengthening community-based capacities to care for orphaned and vulnerable children.

Strengthening health services implies the recognition, in practical terms, that the health of a nation is its wealth. At the macro, or policy, level this recognition requires greatly increased investment in health-care infrastructure, and ensuring the supply of basic drugs. Countries must act to stem the growth in the number of orphans by providing antiretroviral treatment for HIV-infected mothers. At the micro, or household, level improved health status requires more concerted efforts to provide better nutrition, especially for children. This goal cannot be achieved without attaching greater priority to agricultural development, increasing access to markets, and ensuring food security at the household as well as the national level. With school participation accounting for a large proportion of children's time, schools themselves need to play a greater role in the enhancement of children's nutritional status, through both teaching and food production.

Strengthening educational provision implies that every child should have access, for a given number of years, to a school education of good quality. High-quality education, for its part, implies that real learning takes place and that what is learned is relevant to the economic, health, and psychosocial needs of its students and to the broader needs of society. Enlarging and enhancing the supply of quality education and ensuring that it reaches those most in need are crucial to the gradual evolution of an AIDS-free generation in the future[16]—and to enabling the current AIDS-affected generation to cope with the impacts of the pandemic.

Strengthening community-based capacities to care for orphaned and vulnerable children implies the enhancement of caring and economic coping capacities of families and communities. Interventions should provide for the establishment of new community-based day care centers, the reduction of school and medical fees, the development of micro-finance programs, and targeted food assistance schemes. What is essential is the empowerment of families and communities to make their own considered responses to the needs they have identified.

The children of Africa are especially vulnerable both to HIV/AIDS itself and to its impacts. The pandemic attacks their inherent right to life, eroding the conditions needed for their survival, protection, and development. The most critical challenge facing those who seek to assist AIDS-affected children is to develop responses that, collectively, match the enormous scale of the crisis. What *can* be done crystallizes into improved provision for health care and education, improved nutrition, enhanced community and family coping capacities, and interventions to promote the survival of mothers. What *will* be done rests with governments, civil society, local communities, and the international community.

Notes

All personal names in the text are fictitious.

1. UNICEF, "First Call for Children" (World Declaration and Plan of Action from the World Summit for Children, Convention on the Rights of the Child, New York, 1990).

2. P. Vannakit, "Treat Parents and Prevent Orphans: A Project to Extend PMTCT," <sea-aids@healthdev.net>, 2002.

3. World Bank, *Confronting AIDS: Public Priorities in a Global Epidemic*, Policy Research Report (New York: Oxford University Press, 1997).

4. R. Shell, "Positive Outcomes: The Chances of Acquiring HIV/AIDS during the School-Going Years in the Eastern Cape, 1990–2000" (paper presented at the International Workshop on the Impact of HIV/AIDS on Education, International Institute of Educational Planning, Paris, September 2000), 27–29.

5. UNAIDS, *AIDS Epidemic Update: December 2000* (Geneva: UNAIDS, 2000).

6. Zambia, "National Assessment of Education" (preliminary findings, Ministry of Education, Lusaka, 2002).

7. V. Juvane, "The Impact of HIV/AIDS on the Mozambique Education Sector: The Current Situation and Perspectives" (paper presented at the International Workshop on the Impact of HIV/AIDS on Education, International Institute for Educational Planning, Paris, September 2000), 27–29.

8. E. George, A. Finberg, and Y. Thonden, *Scared at School: Sexual Violence against Girls in South African Schools* (New York: Human Rights Watch, 2001).

9. R. Jewkes, J. Levin, N. Mbananga, and D. Bradshaw, "Rape of Girls in South Africa," *Lancet* 359, 9303 (2002).

10. World Bank, *A Chance to Learn: Knowledge and Finance for Education in Sub-Saharan Africa* (Washington, D.C.: World Bank, 2000).

11. E. Stillwaggon, "HIV/AIDS in Africa: Fertile Terrain," *South Africa Journal of Economics* 68, 5 (December 2000).

12. K. Botchwey, "HIV/AIDS and Economic Development in Sub-Saharan Africa" (paper presented at the African Development Forum 2000, Economic Commission for Africa, Addis Ababa, December 2000).

13. Food and Agricultural Organization, "The Impact of HIV/AIDS on Food Security" (Committee on Food Security, 27th session, Rome, May 28–June 1, 2001).

14. UNAIDS, *AIDS Epidemic Update*, 13–14.

15. M. Schönteich, "Age and AIDS: A Lethal Mix for South Africa's Crime Rate," *Konrad Adenauer Stiftung Occasional Papers* (Johannesburg), June 2000.

16. World Bank, *Education and HIV/AIDS: A Window of Hope* (Washington, D.C.: World Bank, 2002).

Section 2

COPING

5

Understanding the Psychological and Emotional Needs of AIDS Orphans in Africa

Alicia Skinner Cook, Janet Julia Fritz, and Rose Mwonya

Interviewer: How is your life different now since your parents died?

Child: I have less to eat now. I have more responsibility.

Interviewer: You said earlier than you were worried. What worries you?

Child: That I will get sick too. That I will have to leave school and will not be able to get a job.

Interviewer: How often do you think about your mother?

Child: All the time.

Interviewer: What comes to mind when you think of her?

Child: Anger. Sadness.

Interviewer: Do you have a memory of your mother that is special to you?

Child: Yes, Mother buying good food, clothes, and paying school fees on time.

Interviewer: What questions do you have about your parent's illness or death that you have been afraid to ask?

Child: Where did Mother go? Heaven or hell? Will I ever meet her again?

The above responses from an eight-year-old child participating in a preliminary needs assessment of AIDS orphans we conducted in rural western Kenya provide a firsthand glimpse of the human consequences of AIDS. Africa is home to 90 percent of the children who have been orphaned by AIDS. As the number of African children affected by AIDS continues to increase, their psychosocial needs are being recognized as equal in importance to needs relating to subsistence, health, and education. According to WHO/UNICEF more guidance is needed to better understand and address the psychological and emotional needs of children orphaned by AIDS in culturally appropriate ways.[1] The attention to this issue does not require new and separate programs but can be integrated into all services designed to meet the needs of affected children.

Cultural variables have implications for children's beliefs about death, their coping strategies, manifestations of feelings, and available supports and resources. Children's cultural background can help define a loss and the factors that make them less vulnerable to negative outcomes and more likely to adjust to their new reality. There may be as much variation within a single cultural group as among multiple cultural groups.[2]

Grief and Loss in Children

Parental death is a profound loss; it can compromise children's normal psychosocial development. Early childhood is a time for developing a sense of competence and trust in others. Children's sense of self and social relationships is being shaped during this critical period and is vulnerable to negatively altered perceptions of the world around them and their relation to it. For older children, core issues related to bereavement include personal identity, fairness and social justice, and a sense of belonging, control, and having a future.[3] One goal of bereavement intervention for children is to create a developmentally appropriate environment that allows children to continue mastery of developmental tasks crucial to their particular life stage. Nancy Webb has used the term "disabling grief" to describe when the grief process interferes with the child's social, emotional, or physical development.[4]

Grief reactions of young children are highly variable, but common manifestations include separation anxiety, fear of abandonment, and the fear that others close to them will die or that they themselves will die too. These fears may be displayed through overdependence on adults, somatic complaints, sleeping problems, or regressive behaviors such as thumbsucking or bedwetting. Unfortunately because of the context in which their grief occurs—the AIDS pandemic—many of children's fears may in fact be realized.

Because they can confuse fantasy and reality as a result of their less mature cognitive development, young children may carry an extreme burden of guilt related to their parent's death (e.g., they may perceive that death occurred because they disobeyed their father and caused undue stress). These misperceptions can be further reinforced in cultures in which the cause of death is not openly discussed because of the stigma associated with AIDS. Children need opportunities to ask questions and express deep-seated concerns.

During middle and late childhood, children become more capable of describing their feelings, verbalizing their needs, and seeking social support. As children mature, they experience a developmental shift in problem-focused coping, and older children begin to recognize they have more control over their environment. Nevertheless, the child's repertoire of coping strategies is still more limited than that of adults because of their fewer life experiences, immature cognitive capacities, and shorter attention spans.

Grieving children will typically show signs of sadness, despair, or depression, at times resulting in social withdrawal and detachment. Although children's experience of loss is painful and ongoing, it is usually not all-consuming. In young children, manifestations such as crying may occur sporadically and may be interspersed with periods of laughing and playing. According to Kevin Oltjenbruns,[5] this shifting back and forth between grief on the one hand and engagement in normal activities on the other is consistent with the model Margaret Stroebe and Hank Schut use to describe the coping of bereaved adults.[6] This dual-process model of grief, in which individuals oscillate between a loss orientation (in which they process various aspects of the loss experience) and a restorative orientation (in which individuals focus on the demanding changes triggered by the loss as well as the activities of daily living), seems to have application to the understanding of childhood bereavement as well.

Grief may also be expressed as anger, particularly in older children, and result in temper outbursts, explosive emotions, and discipline problems as they "act out their tears." For children remaining in school, difficulty concentrating and lowered school performance are common.[7]

Increasing the Risk of Grief: Key Concepts from the Literature

Many factors—lack of social support, bereavement overload, secondary losses, concurrent stressors—have been linked to poor adjustment to loss and therefore to the intensity and duration of grieving. When these factors accumulate they can tax the psychological and emotional resources of children and their families and result in an increased risk that coping will be dysfunctional and have negative consequences.

Available Social Support

The literature on grief provides numerous and consistent findings on the importance of social support following loss of a loved one. Social support covers a range of behaviors and includes comfort, assistance, and information received from others. According to recent research, parental death itself does not necessarily lead to a child's increased risk of depression as an adult, as was previously thought.[8] Lack of adequate nurturance following a loss of a parent seems to be a stronger indicator of later adult impairment.

African families, composing an extensive social network, have historically provided support during times of crisis. In many parts of Africa, practices such as child lending, fosterage, sibling caretaking, and adoption are common, and children have often moved among families as part of this strong and elaborate kinship network.[9] In one of the most comprehensive studies of AIDS orphans in sub-Saharan Africa, researchers found that 44 percent of Zambian households are currently looking after orphans.[10]

The presumption that in Africa the extended family can always provide an adequate safety net has now been questioned.[11] HIV and AIDS, with their unprecedented levels of morbidity and mortality across sub-Saharan Africa, currently pose extraordinary challenges for the traditional African family. Elizabeth Preble asserts that the large numbers of children involved will render traditional systems incapable of meeting the increasing demands for long-term care.[12] New family structures have now arisen, such as child-headed or elder-headed households, and these terms are common in the HIV/AIDS literature. AIDS research has neglected this changing African social structure, yet this ubiquitous disease will

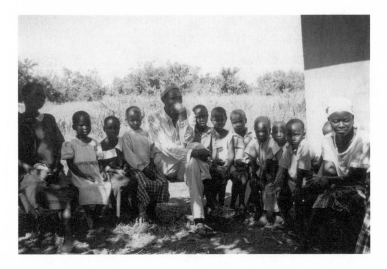

Fig. 5.1. AIDS orphans in a Kenyan village with surrogate parents. The high number of AIDS orphans is taxing traditional African community and family support systems. Photograph by Alicia Cook. Used with permission.

provide the context "in which families are sustained, reorganized, or created in wholly new forms."[13] Not only does HIV/AIDS break up families and communities, it also causes widespread social disruption by claiming the lives of teachers, health workers, and other adults who work with children and families. HIV/AIDS undermines the very institutions that should help mitigate the impact of the pandemic.

Bereavement Overload

Bereavement overload occurs when individuals are faced with many significant losses in a short period of time. Robert Kastenbaum originally used this term to describe the multiple losses many elderly individuals suffer because of their longevity.[14] When children have little time between losses for coping, bereavement overload can result in increased emotional vulnerability. Children experiencing bereavement overload may seem to remain shocked and numb, trying to come to grips with the magnitude of the losses they and their family, community, and country have endured. They may feel ongoing confusion, despair, and a sense that their world is falling apart.

Secondary Losses

The brunt of the AIDS pandemic has occurred in the poorest and most vulnerable region of the world—sub-Saharan Africa.[15] Among AIDS orphans, grief over the loss of one or more parents, although of major importance, is usually only one of many hardships they face. It is difficult for the child and his or her remaining child- or grandparent-headed family unit to cope because the situation they are adapting to is always changing, usually for the worse. Secondary losses and concurrent stressors reduce the capacity of individuals and families to cope.[16] Because children have typically developed fewer coping mechanisms than adults, they are at greater risk of negative outcomes.

From the time a child's parent is affected by AIDS, through progression of the illness and eventual death, secondary losses tend to accumulate. The most immediate impact is a marked reduction in income and other resources. This loss occurs at a time when costs are increasing as care is provided to the family member with HIV/AIDS, and children are often forced to leave school to reduce expenses (school fees and uniforms). By the time the parent dies, even limited assets such as livestock may have been sold to pay for medical expenses and the funeral. These burdens are magnified if the second parent becomes ill.

Concurrent Stressors

Children in AIDS-impacted areas commonly assume much family responsibility. Along with additional responsibilities come concurrent stressors. For example, children often assist with care of the ill family member. Once orphaned, older children may also find themselves looking after younger siblings while still grieving over the loss of their parents. In child-headed households, older children may have responsibility for supporting younger family members. Among survivors in grandparent-headed households, older children may feel the responsibility for elder family members, particularly if they are sick. As one health care worker put it, "In many of these families, it is unclear who is looking after whom."

> After her elderly husband died, Dorcas took solace in the fact that she could rely on her two adult children for daily assistance as her own health deteriorated. Now that AIDS has claimed both her son and her daughter, she has taken her five grandchildren into her home to care for them. As she grieves for her loved ones and adjusts to the reversed caregiving role, Dorcas starts to cry when the youngest child asks, "When are we going home?"

Resilience

While considerable efforts are expended examining the maladaptive behaviors that may result from exposure to high-risk situations, it is valuable to examine the mechanisms by which children come through high-risk situations exhibiting adaptive coping behaviors. Given the stresses and multiple risk factors faced by children orphaned by AIDS, the concept of resilience has great value in guiding prevention/intervention programming.

Resilience is positive adaptation in the face of significant threats.[17] Resilience does not reduce risk, but it allows one to cope with the causes of risk more effectively.[18] Empirical support for the power of resilience can be found in longitudinal studies that indicate that positive adaptation early in life is related to continued competent functioning later in life, even when existing risk factors do not decrease.[19] In fact, children facing a myriad of adversities seem to benefit even more from positive community intervention efforts than those children who are facing fewer challenging situations.[20]

The individual showing resilience is not one who has a stable "resilient" trait, but one who demonstrates a positive outcome within a particular set of circumstances at a given time. A child may show resilience in a number of domains. These domains should be targeted for intervention based on the nature of the crisis and the cultural context. For example, a child faced with the loss of parents in rural Kenya would be considered resilient if he or she exhibited competence in school, provided nurturance and support to younger siblings, or garnered economic resources for the family.

In a review of the research, Bonnie Bernard identified three characteristics (identical for the family, the school, or the community) that are predictive of positive outcomes for children in risk-laden environments: (1) a meaningful relationship with at least one caring and supportive adult, (2) the presence of high expectations, and (3) the chance for meaningful participation.[21] Though a child experiences great loss with the death of a parent or other close relatives, the presence of a caring adult can buffer that child as he or she faces that loss and other related losses. For example, Werner found that favorite teachers or caring friends were major factors in the development of resilience among her disadvantaged group.[22] These same themes recur across various groups and settings studied in the recent burgeoning (and increasingly methodologically sound) literature on protective factors, emphasizing the importance of close relations with a supportive adult(s), schools that provide support and structure, and connections with competent adults within the larger community.[23] Furthermore, research with at-risk families indicates that one's satisfaction with the support received is more important in determining a sense of competence than the size of the support network or the total amount of help received.[24]

Unfortunately, there is still a lack of strong empirical evidence for the role that community institutions and efforts can play in promoting resilience. It has, however, been shown that schools can be particularly effective in providing opportunities to experience mastery and develop important social and problem-solving skills. School-based supportive efforts can go far to buffer the potentially hazardous conditions outside the school environment.[25] However, many children who have lost parents to AIDS often cannot cover their school fees. Efforts to keep these children in a supportive school environment, which can help foster or maintain a sense of purpose and confidence in the future, appear critical to the development of resilience.

Resilient children exhibit flexibility, communication skills, an ability to be reflective, a sense of independence and mastery, and a sense of purpose and future. The development of such skills is predictive of adaptation to later stressors.[26] Resilience can be fostered by reducing risk factors, intervening to stop the occurrence of cumulative risk, and providing new opportunities for mastery.

Programs that are designed mainly to show how to handle negative situations are often not effective. However, most successful programs are designed to help children or adults learn problem-solving skills. They enhance self-efficacy, making children and adults believe that their actions will make a positive difference.[27] Families, teachers, or community members who continue to hold high expectations for a child, despite the loss faced by the child, will also likely foster resilience in that child. Behavioral and academic problems are typically rare, even in the most poverty-stricken areas, in those schools where teachers hold high expectations of their students.[28] Also, acknowledgment of an individual as a valued participant in the family, school, or community serves to foster resilience.

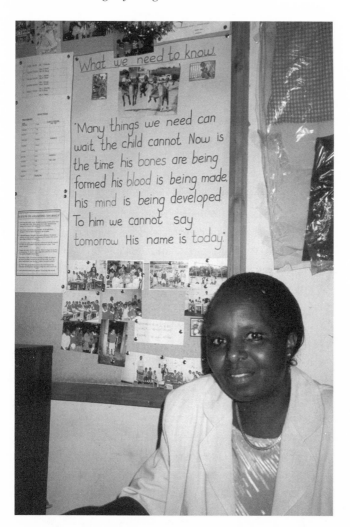

Fig. 5.2. A Kenyan teacher beside a homemade poster. Supportive teachers and schools can promote resilience in children and buffer the negative impacts of HIV/AIDS. Photograph by Alicia Cook. Used with permission.

Strategies for Helping AIDS Orphans

The literature on grief as well as resilience in children offers useful direction for interventions to help children cope with multiple losses. Key concepts include recognition of the need for the expression of grief, a continued bond with loved ones who have died, stability and maintenance of existing relationships, and hope for the future.

The Need for Expressing Grief

Children have been referred to as "forgotten mourners" because adults at times forget the capacity of children to mourn and their need to be included and informed. While at times this outcome is a result of a desire to protect the child, it often results in a child's sense of isolation, a perception that others are playing down his or her loss, and a diminished sense of trust. Children, as well as adults, need to say goodbye to the dying as part of the grieving process. With most terminal illnesses this opportunity is available prior to death, but it may not be afforded to children because of adult denial regarding the severity of the illness. Furthermore, many African societies have taboos about discussing death.

African communities may have additional obstacles to helping grieving children cope as adults are experiencing their own pain and "compassion fatigue." This situation is compounded by the silence around the AIDS pandemic, a silence that Elizabeth Reid has called "a deep unease that permeates families and societies about using a language of sexuality, mortality, or vulnerability" that evokes feelings of guilt, shame, and humiliation.[29]

Lacking personal maturity, children often mirror the coping or communication styles modeled by adults who are close to them and may constrain their emotional reactions in response to parental influences. Children need the opportunity to grieve and have their losses acknowledged. Some children will welcome the chance to grieve orally or through writing. Play can also be therapeutic for young children, especially when they find it difficult to articulate their grief. Play allows children to confront emotionally painful situations using a repetitive process of acting out their feelings and the situations that evoke them. This play should not be discouraged; it provides children the opportunity to exercise some control over the events in their lives. Children who rarely express their feelings through words may spontaneously share them through art and music. For example, one young Kenyan child drew a baby bird all alone in a tree to illustrate his own loneliness. The creative process not only provides an emotional outlet for the child but allows others to see what the child is thinking and feeling. As one local worker shared: "We have real difficulty getting children to tell us how they feel. . . . But there are many signs. When children sing, they sing of AIDS, and they sing and cry."[30]

The application of Western thinking in child development and mental health issues must be integrated with the deeper knowledge of a community's specific ceremonies and customs.[31] Throughout the ages, mourning rituals typically acknowledge the needs of the survivors. These ceremonies help individuals accept the deaths of their loved ones and facilitate the transition of those who grieve from the past to the future. Rituals supply specific words or actions imbued with cultural meanings.[32] Among the Yoruba of western Nigeria, verbal bereavement salutations convey encouragement, concern, and support. They also validate the feelings of the bereaved, emphasize hope for the future, and express a belief in the self-determination of the individual.[33] But in areas of Africa heavily affected by HIV/AIDS, traditional mourning and funeral practices have been scaled back as grieving families struggle with time demands and funeral expenses.[34]

The Need for a Continuing Bond

Children seek to stay emotionally connected to the deceased in a variety of ways—attempting to mentally locate the deceased, remembering past interactions with the missing parent, or keeping an item that belonged to the mother or father. Adults can strengthen these comforting ties by talking about the deceased, remaining alert to the child's feelings, helping the child find the language to express those feelings, providing opportunities for the child to engage in rituals that acknowledge the deceased parent, giving mementos of the deceased to the child, and honoring the child's relationship to the parent who died.[35]

The Memory Book Project in Uganda is run by the AIDS Support Organization (TASO), Save the Children, and another Ugandan NGO, the National Community of Women Living with HIV/AIDS. Parents are invited to prepare a memory book for their children that typically contains photos and information on the parent and her lineage, her dreams for her child, and the circumstances of her illness (to avoid having the child feel he or she is to blame). Sometimes the parent prepares the book with the child present and elaborates on the contents in the process. Other times, a relative or friend presents the book after the death of the parent. Regardless, the memory book serves multiple purposes—it is an important reminder to the child of his or her identity and a tangible and reassuring link to the deceased loved one.[36]

The Need for Stability in Existing Relationships

Intervention programs must recognize the emotional bonds of children and permit siblings to remain together and maintain a sense of connection with the larger community to the extent possible. It has been generally concluded that emotional needs are best met through family and community-based care rather than in institutional settings. A representative from TASO in Uganda says: "We used to just see the child as part of a family. 'Your parents are sick so you have to do this to help them.' But now, we're talking to the children separately, as children, and we're trying to start looking after them before their mothers die."[37]

Preble asserts that feasible, culturally appropriate, and community-based models for child care must be developed to ensure that children's basic needs are met. This will require an understanding of the sociological and cultural patterns of family structure and child care in each country and an understanding of how AIDS has impacted each community.[38]

Peer interactions are important to youth development, and interactions with friends who have experienced similar losses can be therapeutic. Through these interactions, children discover that their feelings are similar to those of others and that their reactions are normal. Peer cohesiveness can also contribute to a strong social network when children have experienced the loss of other important relationships. Older peers can also vent their frustrations regarding the care of younger siblings and offer each other helpful suggestions. Western observers often comment on the strong bonds and deference in the West African peer culture and the child care role of older children. These cultural patterns result from early socialization that emphasizes respect for authority and seniority, and filial responsibility.[39]

The Need for Hope for the Future

Reid believes that "those living within the epidemic, those at the forefront of change, must create a new language that makes more visible the realities of life in the post-HIV era." She asserts that this is already happening in two important aspects of the epidemic:

> Firstly, we are beginning to develop a language of optimism: affirmations of the possibility of behavior change, of the centrality of compassion and concern, of care and commitment. Secondly, we are developing a language of process rather than of interventions, of people as responsible actors rather than manipulable objects. It

is a language of empowerment, of participation, of listening and talking, of counseling, of deciding together. . . . For that which is invisible about this epidemic to be made visible, we must spin the language, weave it into our lives and grow strong in the courage to use it.[40]

Storytelling is a powerful tool for helping children cope with a situation that is overwhelming, particularly in cultures that have strong oral traditions. Adults can tell stories about situations that are similar to the ones the children are facing, and through this process give children examples of effective strategies to deal with adversity. Children can be invited to share stories of their own survival and that of their community. Most important, children affected by HIV/AIDS need to have a voice in creating hope and optimism. Children's participation rights, provided for in the United Nations Convention on the Rights of the Child, have recently received increased attention.[41] The theme of participation was pervasive at the 2002 UN Summit on the Rights of the Child, in which children from around the world helped plan and convene the sessions. Gary Melton has argued that children must be involved in setting the agenda for child advocacy.[42] Youth involvement is a critical component for planning for the future of Africa.

Freshly harvested corn stood in a heap in the corner of Amina's small home as she sat in the middle of the floor with her two young brothers. Finishing her final year of school had seemed impossible after the death of her father and his two cowives from AIDS, but she and her brother devised a plan. With the help of neighbors, her fourteen-year-old brother, Juma, stayed at home, working and caring for his siblings while she finished her final year. Now it is his turn. Together, and with community support, these children are creating a future for their remaining family.

Children are capable of coping with grief and loss if given adequate social and emotional support. In situations in which psychosocial needs are met and social stability achieved, positive outcomes for children coping with this crisis can include increased closeness and understanding, empathy for others, increased problem-solving skills, greater maturity, and a sense of competence. Furthermore, these children can be active participants in shaping their futures by offering their own ideas on ways to support children like themselves affected by AIDS, helping to design effective approaches to AIDS education in the schools, and providing input into solutions to the economic and social concerns that have resulted from the aftermath of the AIDS pandemic.

Notes

1. WHO/UNICEF, *Action for Children Affected by AIDS: Programme Profiles and Lessons Learned* (United Nations Children's Fund, 1994).

2. Alicia S. Cook and Kevin A. Oltjenbruns, *Dying and Grieving: Lifespan and Family Perspectives*, 2d ed. (Fort Worth: Harcourt Brace, 1998).

3. Kevin A. Oltjenbruns, "Developmental Context of Childhood: Grief and Regrief Phenomena," in *Handbook of Bereavement Research: Consequences, Coping and Care*, ed. Margaret S. Stroebe, Robert O. Hansson, Wolfgang Stroebe, and Henk Schut (Washington, D.C.: American Psychological Association, 2001), 169–97.

4. Nancy Webb, *Helping Bereaved Children: A Handbook for Practitioners* (New York: Guilford Press, 1993), 21.

5. Oltjenbruns, "Developmental Context of Childhood," 169–97.

6. Margaret S. Stroebe and Hank Schut, "The Dual Process Model of Bereavement: Rationale and Description," *Death Studies 23* (1999): 197–224.

7. Cook and Oltjenbruns, *Dying and Grieving.*

8. Ibid.

9. Thomas S. Weisner, "Support for Children and the African Family Crisis," in *African Families and the Crisis of Social Change*, ed.

Thomas S. Weisner, Candice Bradley, and Philip L. Kilbride (Westport, Conn.: Bergin and Garvey, 1997), 20–44.

10. Emma Guest, *Children of AIDS: Africa's Orphan Crisis* (Sterling, Va.: Pluto Books, 2001).

11. Janet Seeley, Ellen Kajura, Cissy Bachengana, Martin Okong, Uli Wagner, and Daan Mulder, "The Extended Family and Support for People with AIDS in a Rural Population in South West Uganda: A Safety Net with Holes?" in *The Family and HIV,* ed. Robert Bor and Jonathan Elford (London: Cassell, 1994), 141–47.

12. Elizabeth A. Preble, "Impact of HIV/AIDS on African Children," in *The Family and HIV,* ed. Robert Bor and Jonathan Elford (London: Cassell, 1994), 151–68.

13. E. Maxine Ankrah, "The Impact of HIV/AIDS on the Family and Other Significant Relationships: The African Clan Revisited," in *The Family and HIV,* ed. Robert Bor and Jonathan Elford (London: Cassell, 1994), 23–44.

14. Robert Kastenbaum, "Death and Bereavement in Later Life," in *Death and Bereavement,* ed. A. H. Kutscher (Springfield, Ill.: Charles C. Thomas, 1969), 28–54.

15. U.S. Agency for International Development, *Leading the Way: USAID Responds to HIV/AIDS* (Washington, D.C.: Synergy Project, 2001).

16. Cook and Oltjenbruns, *Dying and Grieving.*

17. Suniya S. Luthar, Dante Cicchetti, and Bronwyn Becker, "The Construct of Resilience: A Critical Evaluation and Guidelines for Future Work," *Child Development* 71 (2000): 543–62.

18. Michael Rutter, "Psychosocial Resilience and Protective Mechanisms," *American Journal of Orthopsychiatry* 57 (1987): 316–31.

19. Byron Egeland, Elizabeth Carlson, and L. Alan Sroufe, "Resilience as Process," *Development and Psychopathology* 5 (1993): 517–28; E. E. Werner, "Protective Factors and Individual Resilience," in *Handbook of Early Intervention,* ed. R. Meisells and J. Shonkoff (Cambridge: Cambridge University Press, 1990).

20. David L. DuBois, Robert D. Felner, Stephen Brand, Angela M. Adan, and Elizabeth G. Evans, "A Prospective Study of Life Stress, Social Support, and Adaptation in Early Adolescence," *Child Development* 63 (1992): 542–57; Luthar, Cicchetti, and Becker, "Construct of Resilience," 543–62.

21. Bonnie Bernard, *Fostering Resiliency in Kids: Protective Factors in the Family, School, and Community,* Western Regional Center for

Drug-Free Schools and Communities (Portland: Northwest Regional Educational Laboratory, 1991).

22. Werner, "Protective Factors and Individual Resilience."

23. Luthar, Cicchetti, and Becker, "Construct of Resilience," 543–62; Marc A. Zimmerman and Revathy Arunkumar, "Resiliency Research: Implications for Schools and Policy," *Social Policy Reports* 8 (1994): 81–17.

24. Jan Miller-Heyl, David MacPhee, and Janet J. Fritz, *DARE to Be You: A Systems Approach to Early Prevention of Problem Behaviors* (New York: Kluwer/Plenum, 2001).

25. Bernard, "Fostering Resiliency."

26. E. Mavis Heatherington and Elaine A. Blechman, eds., *Stress, Coping, and Resiliency in Children and Families* (Mahwah, N.J.: Erlbaum, 1996); Zimmerman and Arunkumar, "Resiliency Research," 1–17.

27. Miller-Heyl, MacPhee, and Fritz, *DARE to Be You.*

28. Michael Rutter, "Protective Factors in Children's Responses to Stress and Disadvantage," in *Primary Prevention of Psychopathology,* vol. 3, *Social Competence in Children,* ed. M. W. Kent and J. E. Rolf (Hanover, N.H.: University Press of New England, 1979), 49–74.

29. Elizabeth Reid, "The HIV Epidemic as a Development Issue," in *AIDS in Africa and the Caribbean,* ed. George C. Bond, John Kreniske, Ida Susser, and Joan Vincent (Boulder: Westview, 1997), 149–58.

30. WHO/UNICEF, *Action for Children,* 36–37.

31. Nancy Peddle, Carlinda Monteiro, Vello Guluma, and Thomas E. A. Macaulay, "Trauma, Loss, and Resilience in Africa: A Psychosocial Community Based Approach to Culturally Sensitive Healing," in *Honoring Differences: Cultural Issues in the Treatment of Trauma and Loss,* ed. Kathleen Nader, Nancy Dubrow, and B. Hudnall Stamm (Philadelphia: Brunner/Mazel, 1999), 121–49.

32. Alicia S. Cook and Daniel S. Dworkin, *Helping the Bereaved: Therapeutic Interventions for Children, Adolescents, and Adults* (New York: Basic Books, 1992).

33. K. Adamolekun, "Bereavement Salutations among the Yorubas of Western Nigeria," *Omega* 39 (1999): 277–85.

34. Ankrah, "Impact of HIV/AIDS," 23–44.

35. Phyllis R. Silverman, *Never Too Young to Know: Death in Children's Lives* (New York: Oxford University Press, 2000); Phyllis R. Silverman and Steven L. Nickman, "Children's Constructions of

Their Dead Parents," in *Continuing Bonds*, ed. Dennis Klass, Phyllis R. Silverman, and Steven L. Nickman (Washington, D.C.: Taylor and Francis, 1996), 72–86.

36. WHO/UNICEF, *Action for Children*.

37. Guest, *Children of AIDS*, 36.

38. Preble, "Impact of HIV/AIDS," 151–68.

39. A. Bame Nsamenang, *Human Development in Cultural Context: A Third World Perspective* (Newbury Park, Calif.: Sage Publications, 1992).

40. Reid, "HIV Epidemic," 152.

41. Anne B. Smith, Megan Gollop, Kate Marshall, and Karen Nairn, *Advocating for Children: International Perspectives on Children's Rights* (Dunedin, New Zealand: University of Otago Press, 2000).

42. Gary Melton, "Children, Politics, and Morality: The Ethics of Child Advocacy," *Journal of Clinical Psychology* 16 (1987): 357–67.

6

Storytelling as a Psychological Intervention for AIDS Orphans in Africa

Yegan Pillay

Hi, my name is Nkosi Johnson. I live in Melville, Johannesburg, South Africa. I am eleven years old and I have full-blown AIDS. I was born HIV-positive. When I was two years old, I was living in a care center for HIV/AIDS-infected people. My mommy was obviously also infected . . . she was very scared that the community . . . would find out that we were both infected and chase us away. I know she loved me very much and would visit me when she could. And then the care center had to close down because they didn't have any funds. So my foster mother, Gail Johnson, who was a director of the care center and had taken me home for weekends, . . . took me home with her and I have been living with her for eight years now.

In 1997 mommy Gail went to the school, Melpark Primary, and she had to fill in a form. . . . it said, Does your child suffer from anything? So she said yes: AIDS. My mommy Gail and I have always been open about me having AIDS. And then my mommy Gail was waiting to hear if I was admitted to school. Then . . . they had a meeting about me. Of the parents and the teachers at the meeting 50 percent said yes and 50 percent said no. No one seemed to know what to do with me because I am infected. The AIDS workshops were done at the school for parents and teachers to teach them not to be scared of a child with AIDS. I am very proud to say that there is now a policy for all HIV-infected children to be allowed to go into schools and not be discriminated against.

And in the same year, just before I started school, my mommy Daphne died . . . Mommy Gail told me . . . and I burst into tears. . . . Ever since the funeral, I have been missing my mommy lots and I wish she was with me, but I know she is in heaven. And she is on my shoulder watching over me and in my heart. . . . My mommy Gail and I have always wanted to start a care center for HIV/AIDS mothers and their children. I am very happy and proud to say that the first Nkosi's Haven was opened last year. And we look after ten mommies and fifteen children. My mommy Gail and I want to open five Nkosi's Havens by the end of next year because I want more infected mothers to stay together with their children—they mustn't be separated from their children— so they can be together and live longer with the love that they need.

When I grow up, I want to lecture to more and more people about AIDS—and if mommy Gail will let me, around the whole country. I want people to understand about AIDS—to be careful and respect AIDS—you can't get AIDS if you touch, hug, kiss, hold hands with someone who is infected. Care for us and accept us—we are all human beings. We are normal. We have hands. We have feet. We can walk, we can talk, we have needs just like everyone else—don't be afraid of us—we are all the same!

HIV/AIDS activist Nkosi Johnson shared this poignant story with ten thousand delegates at the opening ceremony of the Thirteenth International AIDS Conference in Durban, South Africa, in 2000. His account suggests the challenges faced both by mothers and by children who are HIV positive and may have lost one or both parents to the AIDS pandemic.[1]

Psychological Challenges Faced by the HIV/AIDS Orphans in Africa

Demographic projections suggest that by the year 2010 the number of AIDS orphans worldwide will rise to forty million. However, the limited attention given to AIDS orphans is matched by the paucity of literature addressing their psychological problems. The few researchers who have focused on AIDS orphans have found that most develop psychological symptoms as the result of parental illness or death. Orphaned children exhibit greater sadness and worry; do not engage in activities, such as play, that would take them away from home; are more solitary; and show signs of distress and fear in new situations.[2] Moreover, these studies indicate that there were usually few external manifestations of trauma (e.g., stealing, truancy, aggression, or running away more often) but that an internalization of their feelings manifested itself in symptoms such as anxiety, depression, and low self-esteem. However, some children, reacting to the stigma and silence that accompanies AIDS, will give vent to their anger, confusion, and anxiety through self-destructive, high-risk, and antisocial behavior such as dropping out of school, prostitution, uncontrolled acts of defiance or destruction, and assault.[3]

Furthermore, because a large percentage of HIV transmission in Africa occurs as a result of heterosexual activity, there is a strong likelihood that if a child loses one parent to AIDS, the other parent or newborn siblings may also be infected. This means that the child may have to relocate, move to another school, and be separated from his or her siblings and community support networks. Such unexpected loss exacerbates children's psychological distress. Closely related to multiple losses is the guilt experienced by orphans, who often feel responsible for their parent's illness or death.[4] In many cases the normal grief process is complicated by survivor guilt and may result in ambivalent feelings toward the ill or dead parent, including anger, resentment, and other negative reactions to the effects of HIV/AIDS.[5]

Since the psychological challenges faced by AIDS orphans are often internalized (and thus not always clearly discernable), they are often overshadowed by more tangible manifestations of the pandemic, such as health, shelter, nutrition, and social service issues. Given the psychological manifestation of AIDS on orphans, researchers, governmental and nongovernmental organizations, and conference organizers must recognize and give greater priority to the psychological challenges faced by children orphaned by the HIV/AIDS pandemic. If one assumes that psychological challenges require professional intervention, such as mental health counseling, how does one provide counseling with limited resources and in the absence of trained professionals? The answer is not as complex as it may seem. One has to only examine the centuries-old African tradition of storytelling, a frequently used method of healing for the people of the African diaspora and one that could help the continent's children orphaned by AIDS cope with their grief and other psychological challenges.

Why Storytelling?

The oral tradition has been the vehicle for self-understanding and healing since the dawn of humankind, predating written communication by thousands of years.[6] The earliest written evidence of storytelling's African origins is found in the Westcar Papyrus, a document of the Egyptian tales told by the sons of Cheops to their great pyramid-builder father recorded between 2000 and 1300 B.C.[7] Tales and folklore have been the traditional way of passing on cultural values to the next generation. Storytelling occupies a natural role in many African cultures and is therefore a potentially appropriate intervention strategy for AIDS orphans.

Many researchers advocate community-centered, culturally acceptable solutions to the problems of AIDS orphans.[8] Indigenous community-based organizations offer the opportunity for professionals and paraprofessionals who have broad knowledge of local language, conditions, cultures, and customs to create more sustainable intervention projects.[9] When addressing the psychological challenges faced by AIDS orphans in Africa, one should consciously use strategies that are not alien or intrusive. Euro-American psychology is arguably a form of alien intrusion and cultural imposition for the non-white majority of the world, even in remote African villages.[10] Stories, however, provide a way for individuals to cope with group and interpersonal tensions, feelings of anger and loss, and questions of purpose and meaning in a culturally approved manner. Therefore, storytelling would be a familiar intervention strategy for AIDS orphans.[11]

The African continent is constrained by limited economic resources. The best and most cost-effective method of caring for AIDS orphans may well be through community-based service.[12] The portability of storytelling allows for intervention to occur in schools, churches, homes, and other sites in the community, eliminating the need for costly infrastructure. Also, most individuals in Africa have developed storytelling skills. Little training is needed to help facilitators become competent in encouraging emotional catharsis. Even adolescents can facilitate discussions related to HIV/AIDS. And since storytelling is easily facilitated in groups, intervention with many children can be achieved in a limited time span.

Therapeutic stories can be easily transmitted via the mass media. For example, a children's storytelling hour could be dedicated to psychoeducational tales that deal with HIV and

AIDS. With battery-operated transistor radios available in remote areas, orphanages, schools, and healthcare facilities can access the storytelling hour, helping orphaned children cope with issues of death and life.

Another distinct advantage of stories is that they can be translated into many languages and dialects and thus reach a large cross-section of the population. The effectiveness of entertainment-education in the form of radio soap operas is evident in such series as *The Archers* in the United Kingdom; *Raymond the Sprayman, Hopeful Village, Mimosa Hotel,* and *Naseberry Street* in Jamaica; *Ushikwapo shikimana* in Kenya; *Twende na wakati* in Tanzania; and *Tinka tinka sukh* in India.[13]

Finally, storytelling is a nonthreatening strategy. It is effective with children who have difficulty verbalizing their emotions or appear resistant to gaining an awareness of the repressed parts of themselves.[14] AIDS orphans often internalize their emotions related to the illness or death of a parent. The primary objectives of any therapeutic relationship are to establish trust and to facilitate emotional catharsis in a nonthreatening manner. Storytelling techniques allow the child to withdraw from anxiety-provoking material and to engage in a manner that is controlled and self-paced.[15] Storytelling helps the child feel his or her reaction to a loss is a natural one.

Storytelling for AIDS Orphans

Dealing with Stigma and Social Isolation

In Uganda, Zimbabwe, and Tanzania AIDS is such a taboo subject that people refer to it as "the disease," and children whose parents have succumbed to the disease would rather attribute their deaths to poisoning, tuberculosis, or diarrhea.[16] AIDS is viewed as a punishment for promiscuity, homosexuality, and other immoral lifestyles. Traditional healers may propagate the notion that individuals who exhibit the symptoms of AIDS are bewitched. These perceptions add to the stigmatization and ostracizing of many AIDS orphans.

One Tanzanian boy commented, "Since Father died, I have had no clothing and food. Neighbours mistreat me. They chased me away at meal times."[17] A Zimbabwean described the plight of an orphaned child: "Life became difficult for Sibongile after her parents died because she was treated like a slave. She woke up early to do the household chores while her aunt's children were sleeping. She did not have time to study."[18]

It is important to help the child understand that the social alienation and stigmatization is not the result of a personal character flaw, but results from an anomaly in the greater fabric of society. For instance, I have used Hans Christian Andersen's *Ugly Duckling* effectively in a group of individuals traumatized by oppression, discrimination, alienation, social isolation, and sexual abuse. This classic fairytale is a powerful parable that stimulates safe, controlled release of emotions that have been repressed. Children tend to fantasize, and as they become engrossed in the story they momentarily suspend the conscious state, accessing the unconscious or repressed plane. AIDS orphans can readily identify with the protagonist, which was ostracized because of incorrect perceptions about appearance. AIDS orphans find themselves in a similar predicament because of societal ignorance based on stereotypes.

A story can serve as a catalyst for discussion, encouraging defensive and resistant members of a group to explore their emotional angst—albeit indirectly, through the protagonist in the story. AIDS orphans will realize, through interaction with other group members, that their experiences are not unique. Moreover, they will be able to experience their own identities and their problems as separate entities, rather than seeing their alienation and ostracism as being the result of character-istics inherent in their personalities. Through this process of "externalization" children are able to understand that stigma and alienation are the result of ignorance. By this realization, the process of healing is initiated.

Working through Survivor Guilt

Storytelling shares the postmodern perspective of a collaborative relationship between the child and the counselor. The modernist approach to healing, which represents the premise for many Western psychotherapeutic interventions, emphasizes a hierarchical relationship: the counselor is seen as the expert possessing the knowledge that supersedes the awareness of his or her problems, including the solutions to these problems.[19]

Storytelling can allow counselors to imaginatively transpose themselves into the phenomenological world of the child, with the result that the child and the counselor together are able to rescript or re-author the problem stories that saturate the child's life. *Rescripting* and *re-authoring* are terms that describe the process of revising problem-saturated stories and replacing them with solution-oriented narratives. The facilitators and participants jointly explore solution-oriented readings. The following is an excerpt, cited in UNAIDS, from a HUMULIZA peer-counseling session that illustrates the efficacy of re-authoring aspects of the story of a twelve-year-old child who lost her father to AIDS and experiences survivor guilt:

> Her father had died about one year ago. Prior to his death he was admitted to the hospital and because her mother was taking care of him at the hospital [the girl] was responsible for taking food to him [at the hospital]. One day as she made her journey to the hospital it started to rain; people urged her to stop. She explained that her father was very sick and probably hungry and if she did not get to him on time he was sure to die. After a while she listened to the advice of others and rested until the rain stopped. When she reached the hospital she found her mother outside

crying. Her father had just died. She did not express her emotions and became sad and depressed. Since then she started to be very moody—aggressive one minute and depressed the next. She stopped playing with her friends, and her performance in school was negatively affected. She reported that she wanted to kill herself—wanting to follow her father. During the second session of group counseling the children were invited to disclose a secret. Her secret was that she did not want to live because she had killed her father. When asked how she had killed her father she explained that by delaying getting his food to him she had killed him. Moreover, she was convinced that when she was seen in the community everyone else would blame her too.[20]

Some aspects of the girl's story are based on irrational thinking and assumptions influenced by dominant cultural stories regarding AIDS orphans. These aspects required re-scripting and re-authoring to resolve her intrapsychic conflict. The facilitators discussed her father's death with her and the role that HIV played. Other children in the group, who had resolved the trauma resulting from the loss of a parent, reinforced to her that she was not responsible for her father's death and told her they had also lost parents through no fault of their own. By understanding those aspects of her story that were re-authored, the child could access parts of her self that she had become dissociated from and was able to revise her script. From the second storytelling session onward, the girl's behavior started to change; she joined the drama group at school and played soccer with other children.

This story illustrates the multidimensional efficacy of storytelling. By sharing her story, the child was able to give vent to emotions that she harbored for over a year. Also the collaborative nature of the storytelling session—engaging the child, facilitators, and the other children—provided an environment that was safe and trustworthy. Significantly, through the assistance of the facilitators and other children in the group, the child was able to revise the parts of her story that had caused intrapsychic conflict.

Therapeutic Use of the Memory Book

Another effective strategy to reduce the psychological impact of survivor guilt is the memory book, a storytelling technique that originated in Uganda. The memory book is proving to be a powerful communicative tool for children faced with the impending loss of a parent or parents, and for those whose parent or parents have already died. Many households that have been hit by HIV/AIDS are shrouded in a so-called conspiracy of silence. Although adults assume that they are protecting their children by avoiding discussions about death, they are actually causing them psychological distress. Children in such environments tune in to the somber nonverbal messages transmitted by the adults and become confused about how to handle the emotions they feel. Not wanting to disturb the fragile balance that exists in the household, they walk around on eggshells, internalizing their mixed emotions. They become partners in the conspiracy of silence.

Diametrically opposite to the conspiracy of silence is the ability to deal directly with death and dying. A study of two hundred families in the Kagera region of Tanzania indicates that children whose parents talked to them about dying valued this interaction. As in other cultures, speaking openly about death is not natural among African families. And even if such discussions took place, children would not be included.

The memory book, which originated in Uganda, can be used to stimulate communication between adults and children regarding death and dying. A memory book is created by more than one author, usually the parent or caregiver and the child. The contents of the memory book are fluid and may comprise journal entries, photographs, family trees and histories, and other artifacts that remind the child of their relationship with their parent(s), prior to separation. The book may have different sections for personal stories that both parents or caregivers and children can complete. Sections could include favorite memories, family traditions, information about the parent and other family members, and special events that were celebrated together.

The stories in the memory book help the parent and the child integrate the past and the present, and prepare the child for the future. Orphaned children often experience a sense of disconnection from their family roots, especially when they are forced to relocate or are separated from their siblings (or both) after the death of their parents. The memory book bridges the chasm that the dislocation causes and keeps memories alive. This maintains a sense of belonging, reducing the psychological angst of orphanhood.

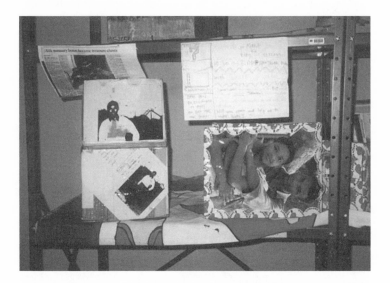

Fig. 6.1. Memory books and memory boxes made by people living with HIV and AIDS at the AIDS Counseling Care Training Center, Chris Hani Bagwarnath Hospital, Soweto, South Africa. Photograph by Arvind Singhal. Used with permission.

Moreover, the memory book can serve as a conduit for passing on cultural values and family traditions that the parents would like the child to continue when they are gone. Parents may make the children aware of individuals or resources they can turn to when help is required. And by teaching the child about HIV and its impact on the family, the memory book may deter risky behavior, stopping the cycle of HIV transmission.

Researchers suggest that the duration of trauma associated with the loss of a loved one is lessened when the loss is anticipated. Mutual storytelling, stimulated by the memory book, affords the parent and the child an opportunity to express their emotions and, in effect, prepare for the impending death. This provides a nonthreatening opportunity to say the final goodbye, giving the child a head start in the healing process and preparing him or her for a life without a parent or parents.

It is imperative that the psychological well-being of AIDS orphans is given increased attention. If their catastrophic situation is not improved, the African continent will be faced with a second wave of infections, perpetuating the vicious cycle of HIV.

Notes

1. Nkosi Johnson was born Xolani Nkosi and was South Africa's longest-known survivor who was born HIV positive. Nkosi did not live to see the opening of the second Nkosi's Haven—a shelter for HIV-positive mothers and children. He became sick shortly after delivering a similar message at an AIDS conference in Atlanta, Georgia, in 2001. He died on June 1, 2001.

2. G. Foster and J. Williamson, "A Review of Current Literature on the Impact of HIV/AIDS on Children in Sub-Saharan Africa," *AIDS* 14 (supplemental, 2000): 275–84.

3. L. Wild, "The Psychosocial Adjustment of Children Orphaned

by AIDS," *South African Journal of Child and Adolescent Mental Health* 13 (2001): 3–22.

4. M. Evans, C. Cohen, A. Shidlo, and P. J. De Caprariis, "Counseling HIV-Negative Children of Parents with HIV Disease: A Structured Protocol," *AIDS Patient Care*, February 1994, 16–19.

5. Wild, "Psychosocial Adjustment."

6. J. E. Divinyi, "Storytelling: An Enjoyable and Effective Therapeutic Tool," *Contemporary Family Therapy* 17 (1995): 27–37.

7. A. Baker and E. Greene, *Storytelling: Art and Technique* (New York: Bowker, 1977).

8. E. A. Preble, "The Impact of AIDS on African Children," *Social Science and Medicine* 31 (1990): 671–80; R. Sayson and A. F. Meya, "Strengthening the Roles of Existing Structures by Breaking Down Barriers and Building Up Bridges: Intensifying HIV/AIDS Awareness, Outreach and Intervention in Uganda," *Child Welfare* 80 (2001): 541–550; UNAIDS 2001, *Psychosocial Support for Children Orphaned by HIV/AIDS: A Case Study in Zimbabwe and the United Republic of Tanzania* (Geneva).

9. J. B. K. Rutayuga, "Assistance to AIDS Orphans within the Family/Kinship System and Local Institutions: A Program for East Africa," *AIDS Education and Prevention* (fall 1992): 57–68.

10. H. A. Bulhan, *Frantz Fanon and the Psychology of Oppression* (New York: Plenum Press, 1985).

11. Y. Pillay, D. Sandhu, and S. Y. Williams, "The Efficacy of Narratives: An Adjunct to Counseling and Psychotherapy" (unpublished manuscript, 2001).

12. R. S. Drew, C. Makufa, and G. Foster, "Strategies for Providing Care and Support to Children Orphaned by AIDS," *AIDS Care* 10 (supplement, 1998): 9–15.

13. A. Singhal and E. M. Rogers, *Entertainment-Education: A Communication Strategy for Social Change* (Mahwah, N.J.: Lawrence Erlbaum Associates, 1999).

14. R. Gardner, *Therapeutic Communication with Children: The Mutual Storytelling Technique* (New York: Science House, 1971); J. F. Scorzelli and J. Gold, "The Mutual Storytelling Writing Game," *Journal of Mental Counseling* 21 (1999): 113–23.

15. J. W. Rhue and S. J. Lynn, "Hypnosis and Storytelling in the Treatment of Child Sexual Abuse: Strategies and Procedures," in *Handbook of Clinical Hypnosis*, ed. J. W. Rhue, S. J. Lynn, and I. Kirsch (Washington, D.C.: American Psychological Association, 1993): 455–78.

16. G. Foster, C. Makufa, R. Drew, S. Mashumba, and S. Kambeu, "Perceptions of Children and Community Members Concerning the Circumstances of Orphans in Rural Zimbabwe," *AIDS Care* 9 (1997): 391–405; UNAIDS 2001.

17. UNAIDS 2001, *Psychosocial Support*.

18. Ibid.

19. H. Anderson, *Conversation, Language, and Possibilities: A Postmodern Approach to Therapy* (New York: Harper Collins, 1997); P. Cramer, *Storytelling, Narrative, and the Thematic Apperception Test* (New York: Guilford Press, 1996); Pillay, Sandhu, and Williams, "Efficacy of Narratives."

20. UNAIDS 2001, *Psychosocial Support*. HUMULIZA is a pilot project based in Nshamba, Tanzania, that functions under the auspices of the West Victoria Development Health Association. It is funded by terre des hommes Switzerland.

7

HIV/AIDS, Children, and Sub-Saharan Africa

Dealing with Bereavement

Susan Fox and Warren Parker

My father died quickly, but my mother was ill for a long time so it was a different pain because I cared for her and washed her. It wasn't difficult though because I was the only one who could give her that care. My mother had relatives but they didn't help and refused to care for children that aren't theirs.

We have to act like adults because no one else treats us like children and we have to do what adults do. Now I wake up at 4 a.m., do the housework, cook, bathe the younger ones, and then I walk about five kilometers to school. When we go to school it's our happiest time because we are away from our problems. I want to finish school and get a good job. I will care for my own children and give them what I have missed.

—Sarah, a sixteen-year-old girl from Zimbabwe whose parents died of AIDS

Sarah's parents died two years ago. Today she and her four younger siblings live with a foster father on a farm in Bindura, Zimbabwe. As Sarah's story illustrates, the death of a parent from AIDS generally follows a prolonged period of illness, triggering many changes in the household that disrupt the child's sense of security. While the financial burden of HIV/AIDS is highly visible in families, its psychological impact on children is more difficult to identify. Addressing the psychosocial health of bereaved children is a critical part of the response to the AIDS pandemic.

While adults spread their love among several meaningful relationships—with a spouse, at work, as a parent, and with friends—a child invests almost all of his or her emotional love in parents and thus has a difficult time dealing with a parent's absence. The consequences of bereavement on a child depend greatly on the child's age and social environment. Children suffer more from the loss of parental support than from the actual death itself.[1] Children's responses to bereavement are influenced by their relationship with the person who died; the nature of the death; the child's own personality and previous experience with death; the child's chronological and developmental age; the availability of support from family and community; and the attitudes, behaviors, and responsiveness of parents and other significant adults in the child's environment.

The effects of bereavement on individuals vary, but whether or not they appear to be affected, the death of a parent always has some impact on children. Psychological damage can manifest at any time, even years after the event, and can greatly hamper a child's ability to acquire skills and knowledge.[2]

Strategies for Dealing with Bereavement

Long-term studies of children in difficult circumstances have shown that they cope in different ways with traumatic and stressful situations.[3] The context in which the traumatic experience takes place is often more important than the experience itself. With AIDS, if favorable conditions can be created both before and after the parent dies, then chances are that a child, over a period of time, will effectively overcome the trauma of separation from a loved one.

Helping Parents to Talk about AIDS and Death

Disclosing one's HIV status means dealing with a number of social obstacles, including stigma and discrimination. The decision to disclose often depends on the individual, their family, and community support structures. Whether or not parents disclose their status, it is important for them to focus on living positively with the virus rather than on dying. The best way to assist children is to prolong the quality and duration of a parent's life, especially through a healthy diet, access to health services, and a positive attitude.

While positive living makes the family's current situation easier, the issue of death cannot be avoided altogether. When a parent is terminally ill, children can sense that things are changing at home. While they may not completely understand the implications of parental illness, it makes them anxious, guilty, and depressed. As children are not generally encouraged to talk about their feelings, they face great difficulty, even when encouraged, in verbalizing their emotions. Using tools for dialogue between parents and children can help both the parent and the child come to terms with the impending death.

School-Based Support Groups

When a parent is ill, children's concerns change and their behavior toward others can also change.[4] They respond to the additional stress in their lives by crying, becoming withdrawn, or changing the way they play with other children. Home-based responsibilities may directly affect their school lives, making children late for classes or keeping them away from school for extended periods. Worrying about an ill parent can cause a child to be distracted in class, or the child can become aggressive while playing with others. The absence of a bread-winner may mean that the family cannot afford school fees, and the lack of money for such necessities as clothes or shoes can embarrass a child into staying home. Without a proper under-standing of the student's home life, a teacher may diagnose newly emergent behaviors as those of a problem child in need of reprimanding.

One example of a school-based intervention for orphans is seen on the commercial farms of Zimbabwe. Families of farm-workers reside on the land and their children attend school on the farm or nearby. The Farm Orphans Support Trust (FOST) is a national community-based program that supports orphaned children. FOST has established Community Project Clubs at a number of farm schools around Harare, Zimbabwe's capital, that aim to equip orphaned children with lifeskills and voca-tional skills and to create awareness about HIV/AIDS in both the schools and the communities. The students and teachers then integrate this knowledge into many creative activities, such as folk dances and drama presentations, depicting strate-gies to cope with HIV/AIDS. These presentations are per-formed in neighboring farm communities thereby multiplying their impact.

Learning Lifeskills through Adventure

Children need more than the donation of food and money to assist them in long-term survival without their parents. They need lifeskills, including hygiene techniques, interpersonal skills, self-esteem, and responsibility. Children can learn these skills through structured playing, which not only fosters so-cial growth and the development of skills but provides relief from stress.[5] Play is also a way for children to work through their grief.

Because of their circumstances at home, most children af-fected by HIV/AIDS do not have time to play, as other family needs take precedence. The Salvation Army's Masiye Camp in Zimbabwe (fig. 7.1) gives orphans the opportunity to learn lifeskills through play. The principle of the camp is the same as that of Outward Bound: learning trust and team building through adventure. At this ten-day camp, children participate in outdoor recreational activities—hiking, swimming, and canoeing—that are contextualized as challenges for the mind and body. Once the children overcome their fears, they can overcome each challenge with confidence and strength. Children also participate in aerobics and running, which emphasize fitness and discipline.

At Masiye Camp children are split into small groups for counseling sessions during the day, complementing the outdoor and craft activities. These group sessions create a space in which they can build relationships with other children in similar circumstances, fostering a sense of mutual identity. Children also learn from older teen counselors, who are usually orphans themselves. Through role play, participating in traditional dance, drawing pictures, and using puppets to share their own stories in a safe environment, children learn coping strategies and self-confidence, so that when they leave the camp, they have skills to build their lives in their own communities.

Empowering Children through Solidarity

Another way to help children become self-sufficient is to allow them to be part of a decision-making process. This gives them the courage to change their situation. In rural Tanzania, HUMULIZA pursues two goals: to assist in the development of the coping capacities of children, enabling them to influence their own situations; and to create an understanding and competent social environment for orphans, which, through supportive measures, can reduce negative outcomes.[6] HUMULIZA has established programs that address the needs of AIDS orphans, including practical adult courses on grieving and how

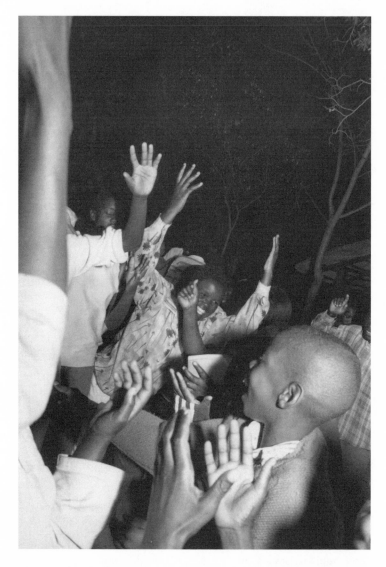

Fig. 7.1. AIDS orphans at the Salvation Army's Masiye Camp in Zimbabwe build self-confidence through music and singing. Photograph by Gisele Wulfson. Used with permission.

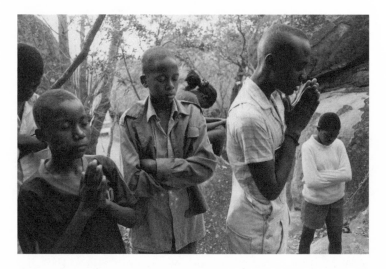

Fig. 7.2. AIDS orphans praying at Masiye Camp. Psychosocial support, including spiritual guidance, is an important aspect of caring for children affected by HIV/AIDS. Photograph by Gisele Wulfson. Used with permission.

to communicate with children, a fourteen-week after-school counseling program for orphans, and Vijana Simama Imara (VSI; Swahili for "adolescents stand firm"), an organization for orphans, funded by HUMULIZA but run by the orphans themselves.

Members of VSI have created their own criteria for membership, including self-motivation and trustworthiness. They have also created their own goals, such as supporting each other during difficult times and participating in income-generating projects. Membership is limited to children between thirteen and twenty; however, younger children may participate in project planning, and those who are over twenty may serve as resources and role models for new members. Activities include doing odd jobs for the elderly, assisting in preparing meals for funerals of other children's parents, even building a house if a member has no place to live.

Lessons Learned

A first step to understanding the needs of bereaved children is to listen carefully to what they are saying. When adults take the time to understand what a child is expressing through stories, drawings, or even body language, they can better provide the love and guidance that the child desperately seeks. Avoiding talking about AIDS and death may seem to be an easier option for parents; however, it can make children feel anxious and depressed and may lead to long-term emotional problems. Talking about the process of dying can benefit both the parent and child, giving them the opportunity to plan for the future and say good-bye.

A positive, enlightened outlook on both HIV/AIDS and death is the only hope for prevention, care, and support in future years. A twelve-year-old Zimbabwean boy expressed this in a poem: "AIDS is all around us, everywhere we see it. Spreading to our family, spreading through our land. But there is one hope for the future, for those who are still young, if we work together we can fight AIDS, hand in hand." Ultimately, the challenge is to build on models that have emerged in the areas that are most affected by AIDS and to preempt needs in areas where the pandemic is still developing.

Notes

For the purposes of this chapter, a child is defined as a person under the age of fifteen. An AIDS orphan is a child who has lost at least one parent to the disease. A broader category, "children affected by HIV/AIDS," is used to refer to all children that are affected or infected with HIV. S. Fox, *Investing in Our Future: Psychosocial Support for Children Affected by HIV/AIDS* (Geneva: UNAIDS, 2001).

1. A. Wolfelt, *Helping Children with Grief* (Muncie, Indiana: Accelerated Development, 1991).

2. Fox, *Investing in Our Future.*

3. K. Madorin, "When Parents Die of AIDS: The Children of Kagera, Tanzania," <www.foundation.novartis.com/children>.

4. HUMULIZA and terre des hommes Switzerland, "Report of the Seminar with Orphans," Igabiro Farm, Nshamba, Tanzania, February 28–March 3, 2000.

5. S. Smith and M. Pennells, *Interventions with Bereaved Children* (London: Jessica Kingsley Publishers, 2000).

6. HUMULIZA and terre des hommes Switzerland, "Seminar with Orphans."

Section 3

COURAGE

8

For the Sake of the Children

Community-Based Youth Projects in Kenya

Kiragu Wambuii

For little Margaret, the sky is the limit. The ten-year-old from the Mathare slums in Nairobi aspires for a life in the sky, as a pilot. One of six children in a poor family, Margaret's hope for a better future mirrors the aspirations of many children in the slums. Her story is part of a collection of images and narration from children in eleven cities across the world, presented at a website run by children of the Mathare slums.[1] Known as NairoBits, the project is one of the programs initiated by young volunteers to mobilize and educate children and young people living in Africa's largest slum on important issues like HIV/AIDS, the environment, and education. The young trainees wish to create a network of youth from all over the world. Their specialized website offers the youth a chance to both share and educate each other on issues of interest. The trainees also hope to earn income by developing websites for interested organizations.

NairoBits is run by members of the Mathare Youth Sports Association (MYSA), with support from international donors from the Netherlands. The association is notable for its mobilization of children from the slums and its use of everyday activities as a forum for youth education. In an environment of prevailing poverty and at a time when the HIV/AIDS pandemic is ravaging the entire continent, where children have traditionally fallen into self-destructive habits like drug use and teen prostitution, MYSA has actively brought together thousands of children from the Mathare slums and given them a chance to get involved in various self-enriching projects.

The Search for Solutions in Kenya

In Kenya the AIDS pandemic has caused a huge drop in life expectancy, from sixty-five years in the early 1980s to forty-six years in 2001. Concerned at the extent of the devastation caused by the AIDS pandemic, governments, formal organizations, and local communities have adopted a variety of responses. Such responses have, however, in most cases been too narrowly focused and constrained by limited financial resources. The battle to halt the onslaught of the pandemic in Kenya in the last decade and a half has also been hindered by a combination of cultural factors born of the traditional African attitude toward sex, a topic not openly discussed. Explicit denial and apathy among the infected and their families have slowed both the advancement of sex education programs and the acceptance of essential basic truths—like the fact that anyone can get infected. Those with AIDS are stigmatized and discriminated against as victims of a sexually transmitted disease. Proponents of the traditional African way of life are opposed to the teaching of issues involving sex, rendering unreliable this otherwise useful means of reaching children. Churches in Kenya consider sex education immoral and have opposed the implementation of such programs.[2]

Nevertheless, there is indication of increased agreement on

social agendas between the political leadership and civil society organizations dealing with HIV/AIDS in Kenya. This has led to clearly visible policy interventions in the country.[3] Beginning in the late 1990s the Kenyan government acknowledged the existence of the AIDS pandemic and sought to get involved through the Ministry of Health–administered National AIDS/STD Control Program (NASCOP).[4]

The National AIDS Control Center (NACC) was established under the State Corporations Act in 1999, following the declaration by President Daniel arap Moi that AIDS was a "national disaster."[5] By this time, fifteen years had elapsed since the first HIV diagnosis in Kenya in 1984. This lack of response reflects the apathy initially held by policymakers with regard to the danger posed by HIV infection.

In those fifteen years, HIV infections increased rapidly. According to UNAIDS estimates, by the end of 1999 14 percent of the population was HIV positive.[6] Of the total number of infections, 78,000 cases were children below the age of fifteen years, and another 730,000 children had become orphans.[7] Given the poverty facing many of the orphans and the breakdown of the traditional system of protection and guidance for the young, most of the orphans are still at high risk of being infected with the HIV virus.[8]

Until recently, the only sustained effort to face the pandemic came from a host of both formal and informal organizations using a combination of short-term educational programs. These included encouragement of condom use among the sexually active and an involved counseling program for the infected. Many of these efforts though were aimed only at adults. An increasing awareness of the pandemic's effect on children has now led to the emergence of initiatives focusing on the young. Beyond these fragmented and short-term responses, there is a need to formulate large-scale, long-term measures in order to respond adequately to HIV/AIDS.[9]

Such responses can fall into two broad categories. The first consists of sex education and awareness programs targeting a particular group. An example is the MYSA program that targets young people living in the Mathare slums. The second consists of direct intervention and patient-care programs. An example is the Nyumbani Orphanage's efforts to offer a home and medication for orphaned AIDS children in Kenya. While health education programs are important in teaching children how to protect themselves against sexually transmitted diseases and unwanted pregnancies, HIV/AIDS drugs are needed for the millions who are already infected.

Sports and the War on AIDS: The Mathare Youth Sports Association

The Mathare slums, situated about ten minutes from the heart of Nairobi, are part of one of the largest shantytowns in Africa. With about seven hundred thousand people living in rundown shacks, poverty is pervasive:

> Mathare shantytown is a stretch of mud-walled structures built on a steep slope alongside the brown-watered Nairobi River that runs south choked with garbage and industrial effluent. And from this shantytown—mostly built of cardboard, rusty corrugated iron sheets and polythene papers—the principal source of income is either hawking, distilling illegal brew, or prostitution. Drunkards, sheep and goats—feeding on the mountains of garbage that are home to mongrels, rats, and flies, and a breeding source of mosquitoes—dot each and every tiny alley and open space turning the shanty town into a huge waste dump—a place not to live; but a place where people live.[10]

In Mathare the dusty soccer fields are an important meeting place for the many young people clamoring to partake in what is undoubtedly Africa's most popular sport. This common interest among the young slum residents offered the platform from which MYSA was launched. Started in 1987 as a small self-help project by a Canadian expatriate, Bob Munro, with the help of local youths, MYSA's principal aims were to organize soccer tournaments for the children of the slums and to help clean up garbage in the slums. Within one year, MYSA's membership expanded to over 120 teams of youths between the ages of twelve and eighteen. Within a decade, MYSA had become Africa's largest soccer organization, with 410 boys' teams and 170 girls' teams.[11] In 1988, after the approval of a new constitution, the project was officially registered under the Societies Act of Kenya "as a non-governmental, non-profit and non-political organization."[12] Most significant, the NGO's first soccer league for children under twelve was started that same year. Between 1994 and 2002, MYSA's efforts brought together an over twenty thousand young people from the sprawling slums and the surrounding area to take part in various community-based initiatives involving HIV/AIDS awareness education, garbage clean-up, and lifeskills development.

MYSA is run mainly by volunteer coaches, referees, and organizers, many of whom are sixteen or younger. Local committees comprising the coaches and team captains run the soccer leagues. Their committee chairpersons make up the Sports Council (one of two MYSA councils), an essential component of MYSA's activities, given the association's focus on soccer tournaments as the vehicle for spreading HIV/AIDS awareness.

In 1994, realizing the ever-deepening AIDS crisis in the slums and its heavy toll on children, an AIDS awareness campaign was formulated by members of the soccer teams. MYSA promptly adopted the proposal, whose aim was to "fight the HIV epidemic by promoting healthy living, teamwork, and involvement in community-improvement activities."[13] MYSA's awareness campaign, managed by a committee of local community and youth leaders, emphasizes the need for young people to abstain from sex. For those who are already sexually active, peer educators stress the use of condoms and the avoidance of promiscuity. The campaign has also focused on reducing drug use among children in the slums.

The senior soccer team—Mathare United—has not only performed exceptionally well in Kenya's premier league but has also represented the country in continental soccer tournaments. From this team, twenty-five young people were trained in 1994 as HIV/AIDS peer educators—there were more than 250 male and female peer educators from all age groups. By taking AIDS seriously these role models send an important message to their many fans both in Mathare and across the nation, most of whom are children. And as a resource for the educators and those involved in planning for the AIDS awareness campaign, an AIDS reference library was established to provide training materials.

Beginning in 1996, by encouraging the participation of girls in a traditionally all-male sport, the association sought to break cultural barriers that hinder an effective response to AIDS in a country where gender bias is still strong. This striving for gender equality in both sports and peer education acknowledges the fact that the whole population is at risk.

Before each game in the league's busy schedule, players listen to their peer educators and share their views on how to prevent the spread of HIV. In addition, yearly training workshops are organized, bringing together many children from the slums to learn about HIV/AIDS. Teams that participate in the training workshops are given extra points to bolster their position in the league. The anti-AIDS logo, which has become a familiar sight in the various HIV/AIDS awareness campaigns, is clearly printed on the association's sports equipment, on the players' uniforms, and on the senior team's bus. It is a constant reminder of MYSA's mission. By integrating soccer and AIDS awareness, the association has sought to make AIDS awareness a part of everyday life in the slums.[14]

Every year the association sends both its leading boys' and girls' teams to Norway to participate in a tournament with teams from many other countries. The association also sends several youth each year to live with Scandinavian families. In both cases, the Kenyan participants are able to share, teach, and learn with their peers from different parts of the world about efforts to combat HIV/AIDS.

MYSA has also joined the Kicking AIDS Out Network, a coalition of sports organizations from both eastern and southern Africa.[15] In a November 2001 workshop in Nairobi participants from seven countries focused on how sports organizations could affect the war against HIV/AIDS. MYSA's success can in part be attributed to its skill in building an international support network (with sponsors in both Africa and Europe), which have cushioned it from excessive reliance on political leaders who, in their use of the organization to achieve their own political ends, may have subverted its campaign against the AIDS pandemic.[16] However, while external funding continues to be the backbone of the association's support, its programs, including its HIV/AIDS awareness program, can only be sustained if the association becomes self-financing. Because of its international success, MYSA's senior team is seen as a potential source of revenue.

A Place to Call Home: The Nyumbani Orphanage

For the thousands of children in Kenya infected with HIV, there is little to look forward to. Not only are they shunned by society, they are also ignored by a government that is still struggling to develop effective AIDS policies. Furthermore, the number of abandoned children has continued to rise as the devastation caused by AIDS continues to grow. Unaware of the fact that many infants who test HIV positive at birth are not actually infected, many single mothers, fearing stigmatization by society, abandon their children at birth or soon after.[17]

Kenya's financially constrained public hospitals are ill equipped to deal with all these abandoned and vulnerable newborns. One institution, the Nyumbani Orphanage in Nairobi, has stepped forward to accommodate a few of the abandoned HIV-positive children. Nyumbani (Swahili for "home") was founded in 1992 by Father Angelo D'Agostino, a Jesuit priest and former physician from the United States who had spent time in East Africa working with refugees. With very little money, most of it borrowed from his friends, Father D'Agostino first offered residence to three abandoned children. By June 2002 the orphanage was home to seventy-six children. As one Kenyan writer describes him, "Fr. D'Agostino is a man with strong will. He will embark on a task that from any point of view looks impossible to accomplish. But he soldiers on and does not relent."[18]

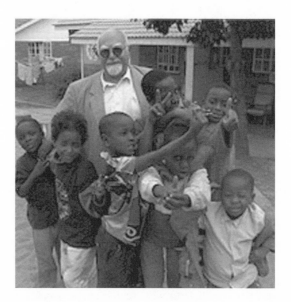

Fig. 8.1. Fr. Angelo D'Agostino with children of the Nyumbani Orphanage in Kenya. Father Angelo D'Agostino. Used with permission.

Nyumbani actually consists of two organizations that work closely together and are funded by donations from across the world. The first is the orphanage, which offers a home for abandoned children until a correct determination of their HIV status is made. Children who eventually test HIV negative are offered for adoption to willing families all over the world or placed in various children's homes around Nairobi. A few are reclaimed by relatives. Such willingness to accommodate these children contributes to reducing the AIDS stigma.

Those children who are infected with HIV are accommodated at the Nyumbani home for the rest of their often short lives. Important for their care is attention to nutrition to build their strength and resistance to infection, medical treatment to combat any opportunistic ailments, and spiritual care aimed at giving the children's life a meaning, while reflecting on the religious basis of the organization.

Determined to fight the usual seclusion and stigmatization of AIDS patients, the orphanage places the children in local public schools, where they mix with other kids from across the city. In so doing, they are offered a chance to live a normal life and to demonstrate that being HIV positive does not preclude children from taking part in daily activities. For example, Nyumbani's fifteen-year-old David O. won a nationwide essay competition.[19]

The second organization, called Lea Toto (Swahili for "to bring up the child"), is a community-based outreach program focused on supporting families affected by the AIDS pandemic in the surrounding Nairobi communities. Lea Toto offers a combination of medical care, guidance and counseling, and HIV-prevention education. Through the program, HIV-positive infants find acceptance in their own communities. While the orphanage deals with the immediate need for a home for abandoned children, Lea Toto offers a long-range solution to the social damage caused by the deadly virus.

One issue that has brought Father D'Agostino's organization to the forefront of advocacy is its pressure on the Kenyan government to allow the importation of cheaper generic AIDS drugs, crucial for prolonging the lives of infected children. The origin of Nyumbani's struggle to acquire AIDS medication is a remarkable tale of chance and determination. A donation of drugs from a well-wisher in Scotland whose family did not need them anymore restored to health a six-year-old Nyumbani orphan dying from AIDS. It became clear to the orphanage that affordable medication would help prolong the lives of sick children.

Father D'Agostino has been outspoken in his struggle to acquire more affordable AIDS medication for his young patients. Unlike MYSA, which has avoided direct involvement with the political system, Nyumbani Orphanage, through its vocal director, has constantly challenged lawmakers on behalf of its residents. On top of lobbying Kenya's parliament to pass a law allowing the importation of cheaper generic drugs, Father D'Agostino lobbied the U.S. Congress to have its members petition American pharmaceutical companies to provide affordable AIDS drugs for Africa. In April 2001, Father D'Agostino invited the speaker of the House, Dennis Hastert, and ten other representatives to visit the orphanage for a firsthand view of the plight of Nyumbani's children.[20]

While no cure for AIDS exists, a triple–antiretroviral drug cocktail has proven effective in delaying or preventing the onset of the opportunistic infections that are symptomatic of AIDS. The drugs do not come cheap, however; they cost as much as $10,000 per person per year in the United States. Acquisition of affordable AIDS drugs in poor African countries has become a main focus for advocacy by AIDS organizations. Initially, drug companies in India and Brazil offered to sell generic prototypes of the patented drugs to sub-Saharan countries at a fraction (about $350 per person per year) of the normal asking price. However, patent holders insisted on enforcing existing international trade regulations.[21] To many in AIDS-ravaged sub-Saharan Africa, the initial insistence by the international pharmaceutical companies that only they could provide expensive patented drugs to the poor African countries was inhumane. Father D'Agostino lamented, "It's really the darker side of capitalism, the greed that is being manifested by these drug companies holding sub-Saharan Africa hostage. People are dying because they can't afford their prices."[22]

Despite the Kenyan government's determination to uphold standing patent laws, in February 2001 the Nyumbani Orphanage boldly announced its plan to import generic drugs directly from the Indian firm Cipla. The orphanage also declared its willingness to accept donations of generic AZT from Brazil.[23] In its quest to import the much more affordable AIDS drugs, the Nyumbani Orphanage had taken the African response to the AIDS pandemic to the world stage. Such a determined stand would strengthen the pressure put on major drug companies by advocates across the world to provide affordable drugs to AIDS patients. And by grabbing world headlines, the action also mobilized many in the world to actively support the NGO's struggle to acquire medications for its residents.

In June 2001, barely four months after Nyumbani's drug initiative and under mounting pressure from AIDS organizations, the Kenyan parliament defied stiff opposition from pharmaceutical companies and voted overwhelmingly to pass the Industrial Properties Bill. This allowed the country to import and manufacture more affordable antiretrovirals. The parliament's move to pass the bill only a few months after Nyumbani's defiant stand to import generic drugs can in part be seen as the government's genuine wish to save its citizens. Yet it is the focused pressure from AIDS NGOs like Nyumbani that delivered a wake-up call to the lawmakers.

Nyumbani's efforts received a boost in March 2001 when the major drug companies agreed to provide previously unaffordable drugs at highly reduced prices (in some cases, free). This change of heart resulted from a significant showdown in South Africa, where the drug companies took the government to court to protect their patents, only to withdraw their petition under massive worldwide support for those afflicted by HIV/AIDS. Currently, the drug companies continue to reduce the cost of their drugs and to enter into pacts with several African governments to offer efficient acquisition and distribution of necessary medication.

In May 2002 a German pharmaceutical company, Boehringer Ingelheim, donated one million doses of nevirapine (under the commercial name Viramune), a medication found to be effective for both treating AIDS patients and preventing HIV transmission from mother to child. According to the Kenyan government, the drugs would help save a total of half a million babies over a period of five years.[24] While the question of distribution has always been a thorny one given the huge number of patients, the government has shown its determination to distribute the drugs widely across the country. Initially, eight public hospitals in Kenya's most affected provinces have been chosen to receive free medication, with more centers targeted for inclusion later on.

Direct intervention for the infected will increase adult patients' odds of survival and will give them the opportunity to participate directly in various economic activities essential for development. For the children of Nyumbani, and many others across the continent, such assistance will offer them a chance to keep on living. While the numbers of those living with HIV or AIDS can be daunting, increasing awareness, especially among children, offers hope for controlling the pandemic in the years to come.

The Way Forward in the War on AIDS

Though both the Mathare Youth Sports Association and the Nyumbani Orphanage are relatively small local organizations, their efforts in responding to the AIDS crisis have had an impact far beyond their immediate neighborhoods and have set a tone for future involvement against the pandemic. In Nairobi, MYSA's example has been taken up by another youth-based sports organization, Carolina for Kibera, Inc. The organization is based in another shantytown, the slums of Kibera. Using soccer competitions to bring together children from different parts of the sprawling slums, AIDS awareness is the key agenda of the project.

The example set by the Nyumbani Orphanage has led to increased attention to the many abandoned children in sub-Saharan Africa and an interest in creating even bigger homes to offer these vulnerable children a chance for survival. For example, the U.S. government has financed a project that looks after two hundred children in Kangemi, another poverty-ridden suburb on the outskirts of Nairobi. The project is closely allied to the original Nyumbani and offers increased hope for the rehabilitation of even more abandoned children. The neighboring republic of Tanzania, also hard hit by the spread of HIV/AIDS, has recognized the potential of the Nyumbani Orphanage. The Tanzanian president offered both land and financial resources to the Nyumbani director to start a similar organization in Tanzania.

Any program aimed at and involving youth must go beyond plain enumeration of good practices; it must offer a road map for the future. If awareness is the guiding light, then hope for a better future should be the driving force, mitigating against irresponsibility, especially in regard to sexual activity. As with the girls in Mathare, wholehearted involvement of the young will lead to exploration of one's hitherto undiscovered abilities and, with this, a new outlook and purpose in life. By playing and winning in soccer, especially at an international level, the girls of Mathare are able to supercede the traditional image of women as subservient. They can aspire to a better future.

Of particular importance is the creation of networks that bridge the distances among young people in different parts of the world. The "Kick AIDS Out Network" has brought athletes together from various parts of Africa and has helped sports organizations push for common policies across boundaries. In its November 2001 meeting in Nairobi, the network proposed a strategy to formulate policies governing the involvement of sports in AIDS awareness and guidelines for the involvement of sports people in HIV-prevention campaigns. Such a united front is formidable as a means for advocacy and is bound to attract the attention of lawmakers and sports administrators worldwide.

Fifteen years after the diagnosis of the first HIV case in the country, a period marked by half-hearted responses and no remarkable policies to curb the spread of HIV, the Kenyan government shifted into high gear in 1999. Although traditionally the state seeks to control and even suppress the activities of NGOs, the Kenyan government has increasingly sought to incorporate the views of AIDS organizations in its search for effective AIDS policies. Given such a window of opportunity, there is need for more involvement by AIDS NGOs and by individuals infected and affected by HIV/AIDS.

Given the government's capability of acquiring and distributing resources, even with a slumping economy there is need to fund more projects to help those infected with HIV/AIDS and to safeguard the uninfected. The government could strengthen currently unreliable sex education programs in both primary and secondary schools as well as continue to import and distribute affordable drugs and condoms to those who need them but cannot afford to pay. More large-scale planning, enhanced cooperation among the stakeholders (both in and outside government), and social mobilization efforts are essential in responding to the AIDS pandemic. At the societal level, there is an urgent need to move beyond the entrenched stigmatization of those with HIV/AIDS. And legislation and policymaking must ensure full protection, especially for neglected children by providing strong penalties for abandonment.

In the spirit of MYSA, which has made AIDS education part of its daily activities, African governments should take the lead in dispersing information and building youth's life-skills. Every political meeting, every village gathering, every presidential press release could carry the message of HIV prevention to the masses. Children who grow up in an environment where HIV/AIDS messages are discussed openly will be better prepared to battle the onslaught of the deadly virus. For now, AIDS remains Africa's most devastating problem. With positive responses, however, this picture could change.

Notes

1. <www.nairobits.com>.

2. John Hopkins University/Population Communication Services, "Adolescent Reproductive Health Needs in Kenya: A Communication Response Evaluation of the Kenya Youth Initiatives Project" (Johns Hopkins University/Population Communication Services, March 1998).

3. The history of state-society relations in Africa is one marked by complete hegemony by the state and outright suppression of groups deemed as opposition. For more on state-society relations in Africa, see John Harbeson, Donald S. Rothchild, and Naomi Chazan, eds., *Civil Society and the State in Africa* (Boulder: Lynne Rienner, 1994). For relations in Kenya, see Stephen Ndegwa, *The Two Faces of Civil Society: NGOs and Politics in Africa* (West Hartford, Conn.: Kumarian Press, 1996), 25–30.

4. As part of the government's reaction to the "national disaster [of AIDS]," in June 2001, the Kenyan parliament, over stiff opposition from international pharmaceutical companies, passed the Indus-

trial Properties Bill. The new law allows the country to import and manufacture the available generic antiretroviral drugs. In addition, the government has moved to encourage increased condom use. The minister of finance, in the 2001 annual budget reading, announced that tariffs on imported condoms would be removed as a step toward combating the spread of HIV. See "Kenya's Parliament Passes AIDS Drugs Bill," Reuters, June 12, 2001, and "War on AIDS Gets Shs. 146 Million Funding," *Nation* (Nairobi), June 15, 2001.

The government also announced a medium-term plan for dealing with HIV/AIDS by proposing a $30.7 million budget in government funds over five years. Kenya has also received pledges of about $100 million from various donors, including the World Bank, to continue AIDS work in the coming years. Much of the money will go directly to AIDS NGOs.

5. NACC was mandated to coordinate efforts in prevention and control of HIV/AIDS in the country. NACC is under the Office of the President and has a chairman who is a presidential appointee and a director who is the secretary to the council. Membership is made up of officials from government ministries, the private sector (including other NGOs), the religious sector, women's organizations, and even organizations of HIV-positive people.

6. UN Joint Program on HIV/AIDS (UNAIDS), *AIDS Epidemic Update, December 2001* (Geneva: UNAIDS). Kenya had the world's ninth highest reported adult HIV prevalence rate (13.9 percent). As of June 2000 the other eight countries were Botswana (36 percent), Swaziland (25.2), Zimbabwe (25.1), Lesotho (23.6), Zambia (20), South Africa (20), Namibia (19.5), and Malawi (16); the Central African Republic had the tenth highest (13.8). See tables in UNAIDS, *Report on the Global HIV/AIDS Epidemic, June 2000* (Geneva: UNAIDS), 124.

7. UNAIDS, *AIDS Epidemic Update.*

8. With a combined slump in the economy and an increase in the number of seriously ill AIDS patients, Kenya has witnessed a dramatic increase in the rate of poverty. In 1972 it was estimated that about 3.7 million Kenyans lived in poverty (defined as an income of less than $1 per day). By the turn of the century, that number is estimated at 15 million, or about 52 percent of the population. See Republic of Kenya, "Interim Poverty Reduction Strategy Paper 2000–2003" (Nairobi: Government of the Republic of Kenya, July 13,

2000). Also, Kenya's Nyanza Province, which has the highest rate of HIV infection (29 percent) also has the highest rates of poverty (63 percent).

9. UNAIDS, *Report on the Global HIV/AIDS Epidemic.*

10. See John Kamau, "Fighting AIDS through Slum Soccer" <www.yaids.org/network/kenya/ken_themes.htm>.

11. In 1996, MYSA approved the formation and inclusion of girls' soccer teams as part of its regular program. Over the years, the organization has fought to overcome the traditional stereotypes of women as incapable of playing soccer and the resistance of parents reluctant to let their children take part in the sport. MYSA's main goal is to increase the self-confidence of girls, seen as an important step toward empowering them to take a stand against sexual exploitation and AIDS-related infections.

12. MYSA Constitution, 2002 <www.mysakenya.org>.

13. For more information about the organization's mission, see <www.mysakenya.org>.

14. Information from MYSA's outreach activities, see <www.mysakenya.org>.

15. According to the figures released by UNAIDS, sub-Saharan Africa leads the world with the highest rate of HIV infection (28.1). UNAIDS, *AIDS Epidemic Update, December 2000: Graphics* (Geneva: UNAIDS). Of the sub-Saharan African countries, the ten most affected are in the southern and eastern parts of the continent. See note 6, above, for prevalence rates.

16. MYSA has received financial support from the Norwegian Agency for Development (NORAD), the Ford Foundation, and the Population Council. The AIDS project itself has received funding from the Norwegian Church Aid, the Commonwealth Sports Development Program (CSDP), and the Strommer Foundation. Also donations of sports equipment have come from Orbitsports. The accounting firm of Coopers & Lybrand audits the association's accounts annually at no charge.

17. According to the National Institute of Allergy and Infectious Diseases, infants born to infected mothers normally carry many of their mothers' antibodies, including the antibodies to HIV. These newborns may thus be misdiagnosed as HIV positive at birth. (These false positives in most cases disappear after four to eighteen months.) Only about 25 percent of those who test positive at birth are actually

infected. National Institute of Allergy and Infectious Diseases, "HIV Infection in Infants and Children," in *National Institute of Allergy and Infectious Diseases Information Sheets on HIV* (Bethesda, Md.: NIAID/NIH, 2001).

18. "An Act of Kindness Can Make All the Difference," *East African Standard*, April 15, 2001.

19. The topic was "The Kind of President Who Should Lead Kenya." See <www.nyumbani.org>, 2002.

20. "U.S. Speaker on Visit to Kenya," *Daily Nation*, April 11, 2001.

21. Cipla, an Indian drug company, offered to provide triple-drug therapy for $350 per person to the international volunteer group Doctors without Borders. The NGO would then provide the drugs at no cost to its patients throughout Africa. Cipla was also willing to sell the drug directly to sub-Saharan African countries at $600 per person.

22. "Kenyan Orphanage Takes Initiative on AIDS Drugs," *Washington Post*, February 22, 2001.

23. Brazil's national AIDS program has gained wide recognition as a model for poor developing nations. Through drugs manufactured in the country, the program has provided many of its citizens with the necessary drugs to combat AIDS. To further advance the fight against the pandemic, Brazil has openly offered to export both the drugs and the technology to willing African countries.

24. "Kenya Gets Free AIDS Drugs," *Daily Nation*, May 24, 2002.

9

Participatory HIV Intervention with Ghanaian Youth

Kwardua Vanderpuye and Janet Amegatcher

In January 2002 a participatory HIV/AIDS prevention campaign was conducted in Accra, Ghana, which reached more than nine hundred youth aged twelve to twenty-three. This low-cost pilot project assessed the youth's awareness and needs concerning HIV/AIDS and engaged them in locally based peer-led efforts to control HIV/AIDS in their community. The intervention employed the framework of critical pedagogy to engage the youth in defining their needs. In addition to distribution of condoms and anonymous counseling and testing, self-selected peer educators were used to reinforce prevention messages.

When her family could no longer afford to keep Abena in the primary school near their village in northern Ghana, they sent her to stay with relatives in Accra. She wound up fending for herself, hawking drinking water on the roadside and sleeping outdoors. Men often propositioned her; and when it rained or she became cold, she went to their homes, exchanging sexual favors for a warm bed, a few cedis, and a meal. Although

Abena has managed to cope with her desperate circumstances alone, since attending the participatory youth workshop she has asked for help in finding out if she is HIV positive.

Adwoa, another Ghanaian, was recently orphaned and lives with an uncle who is raising ten children of his own. Crowded in a one-bedroom flat, she stoically resists sexual advances from her male cousins and their friends. While Adwoa's mother raised her to be a good Christian and avoid sex until marriage, she does not know how to respond to these overtures or the scorn of her sexually active companions. By participating in the HIV/AIDS youth workshop, Adwoa strengthened her resolve to abstain from sex and choose her marriage partner wisely. She has been sharing the HIV-prevention messages she learned with her cousins and friends.

Korkor may be considered one of the more fortunate ones; her middle-class parents could afford to keep her in school. Even after Korkor became pregnant in the first year of junior secondary school, her parents took care of the child so Korkor could continue her education. Two years later, at age sixteen, she is pregnant again. This time her parents decided that Korkor must shoulder her responsibilities. Instead of completing her final year, she will attend vocational school to study dressmaking so she can support her children. On discovering at the youth workshop the risk of transmitting HIV during pregnancy, and dismayed by the limits of available treatment, she summoned the courage to ask about her HIV status at the next clinic visit. Although relieved to find out she was HIV negative, she still has not discussed condom use with her new boyfriend. Perhaps some day soon she will muster courage to do so.

The above are stories of young people affiliated with the International Youth Shelter Foundation–Ghana (IYSFG), a voluntary nonprofit organization that sponsored an HIV-prevention campaign in January 2002. The two hundred young people in attendance at the World Miracle Church's youth service were the lucky few outside the school system who participated in the HIV risk-reduction workshop. Established in 1997 to improve the quality of life for youth from deprived communities, IYSFG provides refuge and resources for women and young girls at risk for abuse or abandonment. The HIV-prevention workshops were also conducted in six junior secondary schools (JSS) reaching over nine hundred youths between twelve and twenty-three years old, the fastest-growing cohort of the HIV-infected population. These young people and millions of their peers outside the school system are the key to turning the tide of the AIDS epidemic in Ghana.

The Youth Campaign

The World Health Organization (WHO) estimates that in countries where 15 percent of adults are infected with the virus, no less than one-third of all fifteen-year-olds will die of AIDS. Even though Ghana is not among the most afflicted African nations, its HIV infection rate was recently estimated at two hundred new cases a day. In January 2002, we started a campaign to pilot a low-cost initiative to assess awareness of HIV/AIDS among youth in Accra, clarify their understanding of prevention messages, and reinforce healthy behaviors through peer-based support.

The objectives of the participatory youth workshop we designed were threefold: to establish a nonthreatening forum for youth to discuss HIV risk and prevention, share fears, and obtain support for protective choices; to initiate dialogue with at-risk youth on perceived risk for themselves or a potential partner, including their capacity to control their exposure to HIV; and to raise awareness of social realities that place Ghanaian youth at risk for HIV.

The World Miracle Church, where the initial youth service was held, is in Dzworwulu, a middle-class community in Accra. Youth services are conducted in a separate building within the church compound. Participating schools, located in three communities of Accra, were self-selected: Teshie, a semirural town of farmers and tradesmen, on the outskirts of the capital; Accra-Newtown, a crowded and impoverished neighborhood within the inner city; and Cantonments, a sprawling, upper-class suburban neighborhood. Depending on the availability of space or need for shade, workshops were conducted in open courtyards of the Teshie schools and one in Accra-Newtown (fig. 9.1). The other schools, eager to give all students between twelve

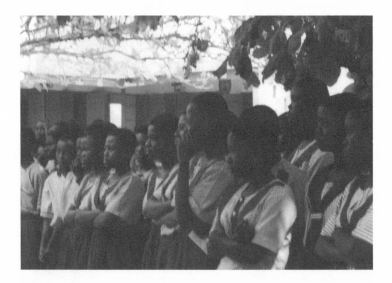

Fig. 9.1. Female junior secondary students in Teshie, Ghana, listen to their male counterparts' perceptions of male-to-female HIV transmission rates. Photograph by Kwardua Vanderpuye. Used with permission.

and sixteen this opportunity, crowded them either into a single classroom, the school chapel, or, in one case, an assembly room equipped with an audio-visual system. The schools minimized disruption to the daily schedule by having every class at the JSS level attend. As a result, 175 to 250 participants and two to eight teachers or administrators simultaneously attended the session.

A Participatory Approach

A quasi-qualitative participatory approach was employed in designing the intervention: the inquiries of the workshop participants' guided the workshop content. School administrators were thus assured that the material covered would be appropriate for the young students. They were also assured that all attendees would receive any information they asked for in order reduce their risk of HIV infection. In effect, the workshops functioned as a large focus group, with facilitation provided by the authors. Data collection methods were informal; groups indicated their agreement or disagreement with several statements by moving to one side of the room (compound) or the other. The facilitator solicited opinions of key informants who volunteered to share their rationale for their chosen position, validating even the minority opinions. At the same time, they provided critical information on risk perception and misconceptions for those who chose to remain silent.

Additional campaign activities included a follow-up to the workshop with the youth ministry congregation the following Sunday—a youth-led debate on the pros and cons of knowing one's own HIV status. One school organized a competition in which students between ten and seventeen were asked to put their impressions about HIV/AIDS on a poster or write essays on how the HIV infection is spread and can be prevented. The video documentary *The Heart of the Matter*, about women and HIV/AIDS, was shown during workshops. Ultimately, the communication mechanisms selected were designed to be participant owned, providing equal opportunity for all to explore and enhance the collective knowledge about HIV transmission and prevention in their communities.

Participatory HIV Communication as Critical Pedagogy

The underlying methodology of the youth workshop is critical pedagogy, created and developed by Brazilian educator Paulo Freire, which has proven effective in raising awareness and the capacity for action among marginalized and oppressed groups.[1] In the Ghanaian context, where the slightest curiosity about sex before marriage is regarded as precocious and premarital sex is considered a sin, the dialogue about adolescent sexual and reproductive health is culturally suppressed. The authors saw this approach as one of the potentially most effective to break the silence around this topic.

In his model, described in *Pedagogy of the Oppressed*, Freire identifies the basic steps of his educational technique as follows: (1) grasp the situation as participants experience it, using participant observation; (2) analyze the situation by sharing experiences to generate meaning; construct and integrate knowledge together; and (3) extend knowledge into the community by acting to change the situation. This problem-posing, or generative, model of learning follows a nondidactic approach in which the facilitator's role consists of creating a safe environment, structuring and guiding group experiences to promote learning. This allows participants to cease being docile listeners and become critical coinvestigators in dialogue with the facilitator, encouraging ownership of the learning process.

To democratize the opportunity for everyone to interact and make a contribution to the dialogue, the workshop structure borrowed from the Theatre of the Oppressed, whose creator,

Augusto Boal, expanded and popularized Freire's philosophy.[2] All participants were invited to declare an opinion through their bodies without employing words, consistent with Boal's "image theatre" technique. Participants were free to express their opinion about taboo topics in the presence of adults by choosing where to position themselves in the physical space, enabling them to override the censorship of their social conditioning. As with critical pedagogy, this forum theatre—which Boal calls "a rehearsal for life"—anticipates that the wealth of knowledge, experience, and strategies of Ghanaian youth would be accessible to all and put to use by the participants.

The Outcomes

As with most cultures, the adults with whom these Ghanaian youth regularly interact—either in their homes, at school, or in their churches—are ill-equipped to converse with them about their sexuality and reproductive health. The willingness of participants, particularly girls, to share their knowledge, curiosity, and opinions in the workshop, was an indication of their courage and ability to withstand peer pressure.

An overwhelming proportion of workshop participants identified late-stage symptoms of AIDS as the "easy" signs to determine whether or not a person was infected with HIV. Less than a handful of participants mentioned HIV testing as the way to determine one's status in the early years prior to developing symptoms. HIV tests are unavailable or unafford-able for most pregnant women in Ghana. This initiated a discussion of transmission from mother to child and the need for future parents to find out their HIV status. One student disclosed that he had obtained his HIV test results on request after making a blood donation at the municipal hospital, pointing to an affordable way of finding out one's HIV status.

Most workshop participants also tended to underestimate a young teen girl's risk of getting the infection from older men compared to boys "her own age." The issues of peer pressure and "Western values" promoted by the media were seen to account for experimentation by teens. Yet upon further discussion, exploitative sexual transactions between young women and older men, or "sugar daddies," were recognized as presenting a more pervasive threat, resulting in teenage girls having five times the rate of infection found in boys. The benefits of creating a support network of male and female friends was broached; youth could then freely negotiate relationships as equals and counter coercive relationships with sugar daddies or relationships shaped by peer pressure.

Most students were convinced that one could easily be protected from HIV by abstaining from sex or using condoms. Most knew that condoms could be obtained from a pharmacy at a price few could consistently afford. Some felt it was hard to be protected and expressed greater concern with all the other implausible ways that HIV could be contracted: through kissing, blood in food, and mosquito bites. Dispelling misconceptions held by students and teachers alike helped relieve anxiety for the younger audience members who were not yet sexually active but did little to allay the concerns of the older students and staff members who were already exposed. The issue of cures and treatment inevitably arose, with some naïvely advocating prayer, others hoping for a vaccine.[3] Most decried the unavailability of antiretrovirals to all but pregnant women, a lack that would inevitably leave a growing population of orphans not much older than they to care for the dying.

Any inhibitory effect caused by the presence of teachers and administrators in the workshops was counterbalanced by the opportunity the adults had to observe a model for dialogue with the students on such a sensitive subject as well as an occasion to get critical information they lacked. According to

UNICEF and UNAIDS, approximately 11,000 of 2.4 million primary school students in Ghana had lost a teacher to AIDS by 1999.[4] Greater measures are needed to equip teachers with the skills to integrate HIV-prevention education into the school curriculum.

Implications for Policy, Strategy, and Advocacy

HIV-prevention efforts in Ghana need to invest more resources in making free HIV counseling and testing, reproductive health planning services, and condoms widely available, particularly for youth. It is important that voluntarily discovering one's HIV status be perceived as a benefit. The prophylactic treatments currently available to those newly diagnosed with tuberculosis (TB) or pneumocystic carinii pneumonia are not recognized as beneficial and are thus an insufficient incentive to ward off what is perceived as a death sentence.

One such incentive was the network of unconditional support cultivated among members of "post-test" clubs in a Ugandan intervention for HIV prevention. Such loosely organized support networks hold the potential for evolving into the much-needed social safety nets for young people to help them cope with the pandemic. The offer made by several of the older students to assist with the HIV-prevention campaign as an alternative to sitting at home after graduation from secondary school indicated the degree to which students were inspired to take ownership of the education and prevention process.

The potential reach of participatory educational approaches, where the target population itself is engaged in defining and sustaining the intervention, has not been adequately explored in developing countries. The concept of integrating individual and community capacity building into the design and implementation of interventions is a novel one, recently being explored in the face of diminished resources.

Recommendations

The model used for this pilot youth HIV-prevention campaign in Ghana illustrates a way to integrate the voice of youth participants in the research, design, and dissemination of HIV-prevention messages. To remain sustainable the messages would need to be multiplied and reinforced beyond periodic, short-term campaigns. A more formalized participatory action research methodology would allow for consistent data collection and appropriate integration and replication of the lessons learned.[5]

Exposing the Ghanaian public to these young people's valiant efforts to communicate their concerns about AIDS would be mutually beneficial. At the very least, their artwork could be exhibited in local spaces and developed into posters and postcards for use in peer education. Similarly the audiotape of the debate organized by the youth ministry could be aired on radio or even reenacted for television.

Notes

1. P. Freire, *Pedagogy of the Oppressed* (New York: Continuum Publishing, 1970).

2. A. Boal, *Games for Actors and Non-Actors* (New York: Routledge, 1992).

3. See Michael Specter, "The Vaccine," *New Yorker*, Feb. 3, 2003.

4. "AIDS in Africa." *African Development Forum* 2000, 98.

5. Participatory action research, often referred to as collaborative research or community-based research, engages community stakeholders in a research process through which they learn how to gather and use information in a cyclical process of reflection and empowering action.

10

How Communities Help Families Cope with HIV/AIDS in Zimbabwe

Gladys Mutangadura

In Zimbabwe, an estimated six hundred thousand children have lost their mothers or both parents to AIDS since 1985.[1] The National AIDS Co-ordination Program (NACP) in Zimbabwe estimates the orphan population to be growing by sixty thousand children per year. This situation demands feasible program interventions. The extended family as a safety net is still by far the most effective community response to this crisis.[2] Traditionally it is assumed that the extended family and the community at large will assist orphans socially, economically, psychologically, and emotionally. This is a common practice in most parts of eastern and southern Africa. In Zimbabwe, traditional strong family ties have been the best social insurance against starvation.[3] These ties include regular urban-rural interhousehold income transfers. When crops fail, family members from the town bring cash and purchased food to rural areas. When a family member in town loses a job, a family member from the rural areas sends food to town for them or welcomes them back to the rural homestead.[4] In an orphan enumeration study in Mutare, all 340 orphans identified were absorbed into extended family structures.[5] In a UNICEF study in Masvingo Province, relatives in the community were found to be caring for more than eleven thousand orphans. Most of the caregivers were grandmothers who were more than fifty years old and widowed.[6]

Community coping responses take the form of different organizational groupings—informal (or traditional) and formal. In hard-hit areas of Zimbabwe, Zambia, and Tanzania, traditional community initiatives such as savings clubs, burial societies, grain-saving schemes, and labor-sharing programs are playing a major role in helping households cope with the HIV/AIDS pandemic.[7] The major activities carried out by these community initiatives include assisting with burial ceremonies, communal farming, provision of food, supporting sick patients, and rebuilding dwellings. Besides providing material support, these informal groups are a major source of psychosocial support. However, as the number of AIDS-related deaths grows, these existing local strategies are under increasing pressure, and policies and programs must be designed that are capable of providing support when existing community mechanisms become inadequate.

Formal initiatives have come from community-based organizations and AIDS support organizations that rely, to some extent, on external support from NGOs, governments, or other development institutions. Their mitigation activities vary from country to country, but include agriculture and off-farm income-generating activities. In Zimbabwe an NGO called Families, Orphans, and Children under Stress (FOCUS) assists orphans in Mutare. The main activities of its program include the recruitment of volunteers from the community to identify, register, and visit orphans who live within a two-kilometer radius of their homes. Orphans are supported materially with agricultural inputs (such as maize seed and fertilizer), primary school fees, food, and blankets. Though help from NGOs is reported to be effective,[8] the number of NGOs and their coverage is very limited. Therefore only a small portion of the orphan population benefits from their activities.[9]

Methods

In 2001 I conducted a study of 215 households with orphans (eighteen and younger) who had lost their mothers within the last five years, selected from Mutare, an urban site (n = 101), and Marange, a rural site (n = 114). The two sites are in Manicaland Province, Zimbabwe, where 1995 HIV surveillance data indicated a provincial antenatal clinic HIV rate ranging from 14 percent in the rural area of Rusitu to 34 percent in the province's capital, Mutare. Both sites are within the FOCUS operating area. FOCUS volunteers helped identify households that were fostering maternal orphans. Qualitative methods entailed focus group discussions with members of the communities at each site and key informant interviews. Quantitative methods entailed administering a household questionnaire to the selected sample. The respondent was the foster parent, who in many cases was a relative.

Results

A total of 700 orphans were being fostered in 215 households. The 101 urban households sheltered 338 orphans, and the 114 rural area households took in 362 orphans. Thus in both sites the average foster household had three orphans. Approximately 24 percent of the urban foster households were participating in the FOCUS program, and 55 percent in the rural areas. The leading reported causes of death for their mothers were childbirth, tuberculosis, HIV/AIDS, malaria, diarrhea, high blood pressure, and meningitis.

Grandparents accounted for 50 percent of foster parents in urban areas and 52 percent in rural areas. In the sample 65 percent of the grandparents were from the mother's side of the family. Other studies also found that maternal relatives were more active in fostering orphans.[10] This departure from the traditional practice of paternal relatives as caregivers represents a community coping mechanism.

A small portion of the household heads were formally employed, and the percentage was smaller in rural than urban areas. More than 70 percent of the heads of foster households relied on informal sources of income. The leading informal business activities at the urban site were agriculture and food vending, followed by knitting, sewing, and cloth vending; beer vending; and repairs. The dominant informal activity in the rural site was agriculture, followed by craft and food vending. However, jobs in the informal sector are generally low paying. The informal income for 75 percent of the whole sample was $12 per month or less.

Education

Of the 440 school-age (seven to eighteen) orphans in the study, 23 percent had dropped out of school after the deaths of their mothers. The percentage of orphans not going to school was higher in the urban areas (70 percent) than in the rural areas (30 percent). The main reason for dropping out was lack of money. The number of rural households with school-age children in school was higher because FOCUS had better program coverage at the rural site. Withdrawing children from school is a short-term strategy for addressing financial problems that has permanent long-term effects that could make it difficult to reduce poverty in the future.

The Role of the Community

As more households are affected by the pandemic it is important to find out whether traditional social support networks continue to operate. Households were asked to indicate the role played by the extended family and the community networks in helping them cope with raising orphans. Forty-six percent of the urban families and 51 percent of the rural families had asked for some help from relatives, friends, and neighbors within twelve months of the survey. The help sought was mainly in the form of food (maize meal, the staple food) and money. A small portion of the households asked for help in the form of clothes, credit, and child fostering. However, 95 percent of the households at both sites revealed that help from relatives and friends is not easily obtainable.

Focus group discussions revealed that the community usually helps needy households by offering them food and clothing and assistance with plowing their fields, but they rarely help with school and health fees. However, according to the key informants and focus group discussion participants, community help was no longer forthcoming because of inflation, lack of money resulting from high unemployment, and prior commitments (since everyone is affected by the high morbidity and mortality rates resulting from the AIDS pandemic). As one respondent noted, "Community members do not have any resources to give to the needy households; they do not have any money or any grain." This finding suggests that the community needs external help to adequately assist households in need.

Informal Community Support Mechanisms

Few households reported benefiting from informal social support mechanisms, such as savings clubs, burial societies, and church-based support. Of the three types, church-based support offered the most help by providing food, funeral expenses, clothing, and school fees to orphans. However, support from the churches is limited to church members, and those who benefit from it indicate that the assistance is inadequate and not consistent.

At the rural site, discussions with key informants and focus group participants revealed that some households benefited from grain-saving schemes, in which people in the community contribute labor in the field of the chief or headman and store the produce for distribution to households fostering orphans. These grain-saving schemes have traditionally provided an important source of support for households fostering orphans. However, participants indicated that fertilizer and seeds are needed to help ensure that the harvests are meaningful and that they can offer sufficient help to needy households.

Formal Public Social Support Mechanisms

The main public support mechanisms that households have drawn upon include the Social Development Fund for Fees (SDF-fees), assistance from the Department of Social Welfare, and the grain loan scheme. However, only 2 percent of households benefited from these public support mechanisms. Focus group discussions and interviews with key informants revealed that support from the Department of Social Welfare was not sufficient. Households reported inadequate benefits, corruption, and lack of funding as the main constraints to using formal public support mechanisms.

Implications for Policy and Programs

The study revealed that surviving children of a deceased adult female were most likely to be fostered by a grandparent. Households that fostered orphans were usually headed by an elderly female. However, the elderly have problems taking care of young children since their work opportunities are limited because of age, health, and education constraints.[11] As HIV/ AIDS continues to afflict young adults in Africa, it increasingly intensifies the vulnerability of the elderly, who are left without social and economic support. This creates an urgent need, both within communities and the state, to think of new strategies for elderly care in areas of Africa hard hit by AIDS. There is a need for a partial old-age support package from the government—one specifically targeted at the elderly, who have shouldered additional burdens, such as fostering grandchildren. Such a program might provide free health care to the elderly, supplemental food, and assistance with school fees for their grandchildren.

The study revealed that children stopped going to school after the deaths of their mothers. The major reason cited was lack of financial resources to pay for school fees. Lack of education will hamper the children's chances of finding formal-sector employment. Thus it is crucial to provide a program that supplies orphaned children with school fees, particularly for secondary school. With a secondary school education, most youths are prepared for skills training and entering the job market.

The study showed that extended families—even though they are still the major source of care for surviving orphans— are under severe pressure, and they fail to meet certain needs of orphans because of economic problems. Informal networks are a major form of support to households, but with the deteriorating macroeconomic environment, the capacity of these informal networks to provide support has been severely curtailed. There is a need to decrease inflation and unemployment, the most dominant problems interfering with the ability of the community to help other households. The government should address the macroeconomic problems the country is currently facing and help restore the purchasing power of households to prevent them from falling into poverty. Only then will households be able to positively help other households to raise orphans.

It is important to encourage replication of the grain-saving scheme, which has emerged as one of the major community social support mechanisms, and help strengthen it through the provision of fertilizer and seed. The grain-saving scheme is not only one of the less expensive programs, it also encourages social integration, which strengthens the community's capacity to care for orphans.

Very few households reported benefiting from informal social support mechanisms. A study conducted by Mutangadura and associates on household vulnerability to income shocks at the urban site revealed that more households benefit from a wider scope of informal activities. The dominant informal support mechanisms cited by the surveyed households include burial societies (54 percent), savings clubs (17), church clubs (16), women's groups (5), informal borrowing (3), and high-interest loan clubs (4).[12] Communities capacities to cope with raising orphans need to be strengthened through these informal social supports.

Foster households were found to rely heavily on the informal sector as a source of income. In a study of 394 households in Bulawayo caring for orphans, 84 percent of caregivers were unemployed or operated in the informal sector.[13] Increased informal-sector activity could play a major role in ensuring that poor households have a source of income. In my study, the informal activities that were mostly used by households to cope were vending, agriculture, crafts, and sewing/knitting. The level of output and earnings in the informal sector can be increased by enacting policies that improve access to financing, create a supportive regulatory environment and supportive infrastructure, remove prohibitive by-laws hindering the operations of the informal sector, ensure training, and disseminate information about appropriate technologies.[14]

Notes

1. UNAIDS, *AIDS Epidemic Update: December 2000* (Geneva: UNAIDS, 2000).

2. C. Mukoyogo and G. Williams, "AIDS Orphans: A Community Perspective from Tanzania," *Strategies for Hope* 5 (1991).

3. C. B. Thompson, "Drought Management in Southern Africa: From Relief through Rehabilitation to Vulnerability Reduction" (Report prepared in association with the SADC Food Security Unit for UNICEF, Harare, 1993).

4. Ibid.

5. G. Foster, R. Shakespeare, F. Chinemana, H. Jackson, S. Gregson, C. Marange, and S. Mashumba, "Orphan Prevalence and Extended Family Care in a Peri-Urban Community in Zimbabwe," *AIDS Care* 7 (1995): 3–17.

6. UNAIDS, *Children Orphaned by AIDS: Frontline Responses from Eastern and Southern Africa* (Geneva: UNAIDS, 1999).

7. G. Mutangadura, E. Makaudze, D. Mukurazita, and H. Jackson, *A Review of Household and Community Responses to the HIV/AIDS Epidemic in the Rural Areas of Sub-Saharan Africa* (Geneva: UNAIDS, 1999); E. Kaseke, *Social Security Systems in Rural Zimbabwe* (Harare: Friedrich Ebert Stiftung, 1997).

8. G. Mutangadura and E. Makaudze, "Urban Vulnerability to Income Shocks and Effectiveness of Current Social Protection Mechanisms: The Case of Zimbabwe" (Consultancy Report for the Ministry of Public Service, Labor and Social Welfare and the World Bank, 2000).

9. R. Drew, G. Foster, and J. Chitima, "Cultural Practices of Orphaned Families in the North Nyanga District of Zimbabwe," *Journal of Social Development in Africa* 11 (1996): 79–86.

10. Foster et al., "Orphan Prevalence"; M. Urassa, J. T. Boerma, J. Z. L. Ng'weshemi, R. Isingo, D. Schapink, and Y. Kumogola, "Orphanhood, Child Fostering, and the AIDS Epidemic in Rural Tanzania," *Health Transition Review* 7 (supplement 2) (1997): 141–53.

11. Foster et al., "Orphan Prevalence."

12. Mutangadura and Makaudze, "Urban Vulnerability."

13. J. Mthombeni and S. German, "Children of the Cities: A Situation Analysis of Urban Orphans Due to AIDS in Bulawayo" (12th World AIDS Conference, Bridging the Gap, Geneva, June 28–July 3, 1998).

14. Mutangadura and Makaudze, "Urban Vulnerability."

Section 4

POSSIBILITY

11

Sara: A Role Model for African Girls Facing HIV/AIDS

Neill McKee, with Mira Aghi,
Rachel Carnegie, and Nuzhat Shahzadi

One of the fundamental causes of the spread of HIV/AIDS in sub-Saharan Africa is gender inequality within a context of income disparity and poverty.[1] Not only are females biologically more susceptible than males to infection with HIV,[2] they are more at risk because of sociocultural conditioning.[3] In many parts of Africa, the manifestations of this inequality can be seen at an early age. Girls have fewer opportunities than boys. They are seen primarily as future child bearers and nurturers.[4] At an early age girls are socialized to perform subservient roles. When older, they often lack crucial psychosocial skills, such as the ability to communicate assertively, to think critically, to make decisions and negotiate, to solve problems in social relationships, to resist pressure, and to cope with emotions and conflict.[5] African girls enter into relationships with the opposite sex as unequal partners. Many interventions and much research have focused on adolescents, yet the gender-based socialization of boys and girls continues to create unequal power in sexual relationships, putting young women at a disadvantage.[6] This has grave implications for young girls, given the rapid spread of HIV.

In 1994, UNICEF decided that in order to support other programs for the fulfillment of the rights of children to survival, protection, and development, a far-reaching, regional communication strategy was required. The Sara Communication Initiative (SCI) was designed as a set of communication tools that would fit UNICEF's own programs and those of other partner organizations.[7] The complexity of factors required for behavior change and positive behavior development warranted a multimedia, entertainment-education approach[8] that would capture the imagination and attention of adolescent girls and be acceptable to their male peers and their parents. With proper formative research, a set of characters, backgrounds, and story lines could be designed in animated film and comic book formats that would "strike a common chord" across eastern and southern Africa—a large region with diverse cultures. Later, the same materials were tested and introduced successfully in Nigeria, Ivory Coast, and Ghana.

UNICEF concluded that both animated film in video format and comic books could be used as regional communication tools to communicate difficult social issues, portraying them in sensitive, nonthreatening ways without losing message impact.[9] Sara's creators built on the experience of Meena (a young South Asian girl), UNICEF communication initiative in South Asia that started in 1991 and that has popularized a dynamic, younger role model who stands for gender equity and the rights of female children. Meena, widely popular in South Asia, continues to be used by local partners to change discriminatory attitudes and behavior toward girls.[10]

The Sara stories had to address a range of factors that influence the behavior of African adolescents (from ten to nineteen). Stories had to be informative while motivating people to change; they also had to address the skills to act, while reflecting environmental factors that might facilitate or impede positive change.[11] In addition to broadcasting Sara videos and a radio series, the use of Sara print materials in formal and informal educational settings was deemed equally important. It was recognized that group processes, including interactive learning methods, are required to develop psychosocial lifeskills.[12] With gender inequality driving the HIV/AIDS pandemic in Africa, the challenge for the SCI creators was formidable.[13]

Sara Themes and Stories

Based on UNICEF's regional priorities and the needs identified in communities, the SCI involved the development of communication tools to address the causes of HIV/AIDS. Although most efforts in HIV/AIDS prevention in the mid-1990s were focused on older, so-called high-risk groups, the Sara team believed that adolescents in sub-Saharan Africa were at great risk and that interventions should begin at a young age. Because they had an unequal start in life, girls in particular had to be empowered. The first Sara story, "The Special Gift," suggested that educating girls and keeping them in safe school environments protects them from HIV.[14] In addition, it provided a role model for teachers, emphasizing their responsibility for protecting girls from sexual exploitation.

The subsequent Sara stories centered on the causes and outcomes of HIV/AIDS, emphasizing the impact of the pandemic on adolescent girls. However, as didactic messages about HIV/AIDS could be counterproductive, a subtle approach was taken in developing the Sara materials. Subsequent Sara stories included "Sara Saves Her Friend," focusing on sexual abuse and exploitation; "Daughter of a Lioness," dealing with female genital cutting (which contributes to HIV infections) and gender role socialization; "The Trap," dealing with sexual exploitation by "sugar daddies"; "Choices," highlighting the consequences of teenage pregnancy; "The Empty Compound," emphasizing the importance of breaking the silence on HIV/ AIDS and care and support for orphans; "Who Is the Thief?" dealing with child labor and sexual exploitation in urban areas; and "Sara and the Boy Soldier," focusing on the protection of adolescent girls during civil conflict and war (fig. 11.1).

Addressing young adolescents, particularly girls, as a main audience in HIV/AIDS prevention appears to be important. In Uganda, where HIV incidence has declined substantially, the accumulated work of many community-based, faith-based, and media-based initiatives has helped to increase the age of sexual debut and reduce the average number of sexual partners of young people.[15] In Uganda programs aimed at young people— particularly girls—helped build their skills to resist unwanted sex and led to the setting of community norms through the mass media and interpersonal and community channels.

Recognizing that any proposed changes in girls' lives would have to be supported by boys and parents the creators of Sara involved them in the research and creation of their stories. Male and female characters of different ages serve as protagonists or antagonists for the cause of girls' rights (fig. 11.2). The modeling of positive gender relations starting at an early age, was especially important. So Sara's friend Juma, his older brother, and Sara's father and younger brother all play key, positive roles in her life. For example, in "The Trap" Juma and his older brother help Sara ward off sexual harassment by an older man. In "Daughter of a Lioness" Juma helps Sara get away from the ceremony for female genital cutting. In "The Special Gift" Sara's father strongly supports her right to education, while her younger brother provides emotional support.

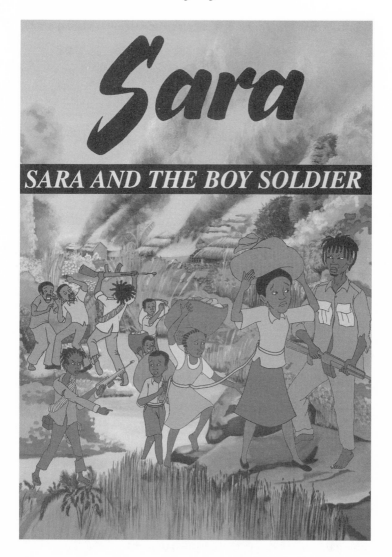

Fig. 11.1. Cover of the comic book *Sara and the Boy Soldier.* Sara is second from the right. UNICEF.

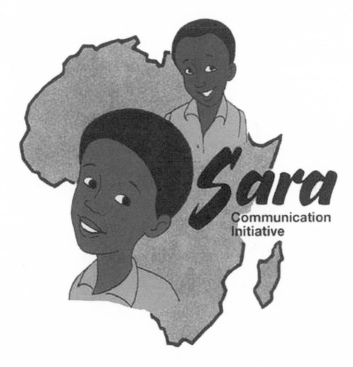

Fig. 11.2. Sara (foreground) with her brother, the protagonists of the Sara Communication Initiative. UNICEF.

The Formative Research Process

The formative research process, the foundation of the SCI, began in October 1994 through a participatory consultation in Machakos, Kenya, with over sixty researchers, writers, and health and gender specialists from ten African countries.[16] This consultation led to the development of the Sara story themes, plot lines, characters, and their names. Subsequently, in two subregional workshops, researchers were trained to carry out a common research process in their own countries. For the pilot phase during 1995, 572 focus group discussions were conducted with over five thousand respondents in ten eastern and southern African countries. Nigeria, Ivory Coast, and Ghana were added later. Approximately three thousand more respondents were included in subsequent research. The formative research involved girls and boys (ages twelve to eighteen) and their mothers, fathers, or guardians, as well as key members of the community. This massive undertaking provided a holistic understanding of the social pressures put on girls, which contribute to their vulnerability.

Formative research also established the names, attributes, and appearance of the cast of Sara characters, including the protagonist. The name Sara was found to be acceptable in both Christian and Muslim communities across Africa. The other names on the short list were given to Sara's family and friends. Formative research was carried out on two to three stories at a time by the national research teams. The research processed followed three cycles: first, concept testing, to understand perceptions of a specific educational issue; second, research on a draft story line; finally, testing on the revised story with color illustrations. The researchers examined each story's entertainment value, relevance to local situations, credibility, realism, clarity, comprehension, characterization, cultural acceptability, potential to stimulate discussion, and potential impact. The illustrations of the characters and locales in each country were checked for suitability.

The national research teams produced detailed reports at each stage. Each cycle of research concluded with a regional workshop in which the researchers, writers, and artists met to discuss the research findings, further refining the stories and designs. Formative research helped the creators of the SCI gauge how communities perceived problems relating to the exploitation of the girl child, including identifying solutions that were credible and achievable. During the research process, the respondents themselves became partners in the creation of the stories.[17]

The pilot package for episode one—a Sara video, comic book, posters, radio series, and users' guide—was assessed for acceptability in eleven countries: Ethiopia, Ivory Coast, Kenya, Malawi, Mozambique, Namibia, Nigeria, South Africa, Tanzania, Zambia, and Zimbabwe. In each country, the research teams conducted fourteen to twenty focus group discussions among respondents in different cultural and urban/rural settings. The purpose was to assess whether adolescent girls are motivated and encouraged by Sara's experiences, whether they identify with Sara, and how the community members accept the stands taken by Sara. The research results on the pilot package led to the following conclusion:

> Sara was seen as a universally acceptable, entertaining symbol for the adolescent girl throughout the region. The story and its objectives were well understood. Sara was seen as a credible source of education on the themes. Most audiences consider the situations portrayed as real. The use of animation does not distract from the reality that the story puts forward. Sara was seen as a daughter or the girl next door in diverse cultures. The characters are acceptable in all cultures, including the animals that are seen as thematically intrinsic to the stories. The Sara materials were viewed by target groups as having great potential for behavioral change and behavioral development of children. The story not only describes the situation of girls in Africa, it offers realistic solutions.[18]

The results of the pilot testing were fed back into the development of subsequent Sara materials. Each video episode of the Sara series followed a similar research process to ensure quality and relevance.

Formative Research for "Choices"

The "Choices" episode addressed several educational issues: trying to avoid teenage pregnancy and coping with its consequences when it occurs; school-age mothers returning to school; developing positive relationships between boys and girls through modeling lifeskills, including resisting peer pressure; and coping with stress and emotions.

The main plot follows the story of Sara's friend Tamala, who is impregnated by Sara's cousin Jackson. Jackson believes that to prove his manhood he has to have sex with girls. But he refuses to share the responsibility for Tamala's pregnancy. Sara discovers Tamala's problem and helps her. The subplot reveals Sara's own emotions toward Musa, an older boy, who is in love with her. Pressured by his peers, Musa tries to push Sara into having sex with him (fig. 11.3). Although she likes Musa, Sara is shocked by his behavior and rejects his advances. The story reaches its climax when Jackson, afraid to face his father, tries to run away across a flooded river and almost drowns. Sara and Musa, together, help Jackson out of the river, and he decides to return to his village and face the consequences of his relationship with Tamala. Jackson's father agrees to pay for the maintenance of Tamala and the baby. With her teacher's support, Tamala returns to another school after the baby's

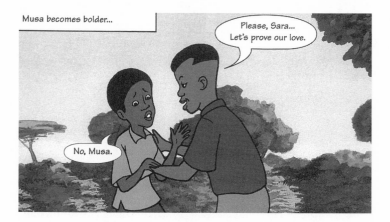

Fig. 11.3. A scene from the comic book *Choices* in which Musa tries to force himself on Sara. UNICEF.

birth. Sara and Musa also work out a mutually respectful way to proceed with their relationship.

The formative research process led to fine-tuning the characterizations of the various protagonists to enhance their credibility with an adolescent audience. The process showed that

- Sara needed to show more vulnerability and human emotion in her relationship with Musa.
- Musa needed to show greater internal conflict so that his inappropriate behavior was more understandable and his regret more credible. Only then would the target audience believe that his relationship with Sara might have a future.
- Tamala's character needed to be made more likable so that she could evoke greater empathy. Also, audience members wished to see her as being wiser after her experience.
- Jackson needed to be further exposed for his weakness and hypocrisy. Audience members wanted him to be unfavorably contrasted with a reformed Musa so that he would not become an antihero for adolescent boys.

Pretesting showed that the near-final version of the story, with the above refinements, strongly communicated the educational issues, but it still scored low on dramatic content. The storm scene and Jackson's harrowing rescue from river waters were added to build dramatic tension, and to provide Jackson a reason to reflect on his actions.

Program Implementation

In mid-1996, Sara was launched through a thirteen-episode radio drama series in English, French, Hausa, Swahili, and Portuguese. The radio series was produced in collaboration with the BBC World Service and broadcast across Africa. The radio broadcasts led to the official launch on September 13, 1996, at the Organisation of African Unity's Conference on the Empowerment of Women through Functional Literacy and the Education of the Girl Child, held in Kampala, Uganda. Over the next five years (1996–2001), episodes two through eight of Sara were completed, involving the same artists, writers, and communication researchers from the region. All participating countries were helped by the regional Sara team to disseminate materials through mass media, government, NGO, and commercial channels. The following spectrum of activities were carried out in implementation countries:

- national training workshops on the use of Sara materials
- development of local Sara materials
- formation of core Sara groups for dissemination and utilization
- wide use of Sara materials by government partners and NGOs
- training of facilitators for effective utilization
- establishment of Sara clubs and peer educator programs
- distribution of Sara materials to schools
- broadcast of Sara videos on national television networks
- rebroadcast of the Sara radio series on national stations
- local-language translations of materials
- screening of Sara videos to audiences through video outreach systems
- training of local artists and writers
- Sara advocacy festivals[19]

The Sara Communication Initiative did not function as a single, centralized project with an overseeing director. Since UNICEF is set up as a decentralized, country-based organization, regional communication projects are unusual. Therefore, no country was required to devote human and financial resources to use Sara materials. Utilization depended on the ability of the Sara teams in each country, with support from the regional team, to integrate the concept and materials into new and existing programs. As the problem of adolescent girls are similar throughout sub-Saharan Africa, and as Sara materials were developed in a regional context, several countries found them to be relevant and cost-effective.

The Mid-Term Evaluation

A mid-term evaluation for Sara was conducted by independent research experts (results are summarized below).[20] The first component of the SCI evaluation was a study of the implementation process itself. By documenting the differences in the way the SCI was implemented in different countries, the variations in project outcomes could perhaps be explained. Since the SCI was not a stand-alone project but depended on integration in UNICEF country programs, the main questions guiding the evaluation study were: How have UNICEF policies influenced the implementation of the SCI? How has the UNICEF country program's acceptance of the SCI influenced its implementation? How has UNICEF worked with intersectoral partners to implement the SCI?

In a number of countries the demand for and impact of Sara materials was tremendous. In other countries UNICEF and its partners were slow in adopting the Sara materials. The following key elements were identified for the success of Sara: (1) An enabling environment within UNICEF country offices, with strong leadership providing support for the SCI, including a forceful advocate for Sara within UNICEF to move the program forward. The interest and influence of the UNICEF country representative was especially important. (2) The SCI was intensely adopted where the people responsible for Sara in each UNICEF office did effective internal marketing to gain support across different program sections. (3) The SCI was especially effective in countries where there was a broad sense of ownership of the program, where the implementing partners felt that the initiative belonged to them.

The second component of the evaluation was a study of outcomes, with both quantitative and qualitative components. Since undertaking statistical research in all implementation countries was expensive, it was decided to purposively choose a country where the SCI had been used widely, as intended, in order to determine its overall impact. A sample survey was conducted in twenty-five districts of mainland Tanzania, where the SCI had been implemented for two years. Mbago and Sichona found that out of 635 girls interviewed, 32 percent could correctly identify Sara when shown an illustration of her; 18 percent said they had read the comic books, and 15 percent had shared a story with others. Ten percent of the respondents had heard about Sara through the radio show; 15 percent had seen a Sara video; and 9 percent recalled a Sara poster. After only two years of programming, Sara was identified correctly by one-third of the girls in these districts of Tanzania.[21]

The third component of the evaluation was a qualitative study of the SCI outcomes in Kenya and Uganda. This study was conducted to provide insights about the role of the SCI in changing attitude and behaviors, especially in assessing how Sara influenced the development of lifeskills among girls. An attempt was also made to determine how well the Sara materials were incorporated into the programs of different organizations. The research involved discussions with users, in-depth interviews, and focus group discussions (FGDs) with girls who were well exposed to Sara through educational processes, usually with trained facilitators. The present analysis is restricted to a content analysis of data with direct reference to:

(1) sexual harassment and abuse, and (2) perception of Sara as a role model for girls.

A focus group discussion in an urban setting—a drop-in center for street children in Nairobi—demonstrated how children are applying Sara's experiences and behavior in their lives while still being acutely aware of their own difficult circumstances.[22] The research revealed a range of lifeskills being developed, including risk assessment and critical thinking. The adolescents were able to relate the Sara materials to real-life situations. They talked about their own encounters with truck drivers, for instance. They said that girls should learn to say no to the sexual advances from older men. While Sara emerged as the respondents' favorite character, some thought she was rather green—in reality, most girls living on the street are sexually active and experienced. Teachers noted that the girls were inspired by the character of Sara, as she reassured them of their own abilities.

In Uganda qualitative research was carried out with girls who attend school.[23] In one area of Uganda nine key informant interviews and five FGDs were carried out with members of lifeskills clubs, established by the Forum of African Women Educationists (FAWE). Of the sixty-three lifeskills clubs operating in six districts in 2000, Nuwagaba and Neema randomly selected Mukono District.[24] Two schools in Mukono District were selected that were mixed (where gender relations could be assessed) and that had functional lifeskills clubs. Respondents for key informant interviews had to be of various ages between ten and nineteen, from different peer groups, and must have been exposed to the SCI and lifeskills through group work. The respondents were shown an image of Sara and were asked if they knew her name. In all cases the girls knew Sara. When they were asked what kind of a girl Sara was, the following responses were compiled:

Sara is an adolescent girl; Sara is the cleverest girl in the world; Sara is a girl who set her eyes on higher education; Sara gives advice to her friends; Sara is a critical thinker; If you know about Sara, you will never have any problem that you cannot solve; Sara is our *Bible*; Sara is a girl who solves problems; and so on. (emphasis added)

A comment from FGDs at Mukono High School gives more insight into Sara's role in resolving relationship problems with boys who pressure girls to have sex:

A boy whom we study with at school came and exactly told me that same thing as we learnt in Sara lifeskills club. He said that even if it meant dying, he was determined to die for me because of his great passion toward me. His words seemed so sweet but that good heart inside me kept haunting me, saying, "Do you remember what you learnt in Sara and the lifeskills club?" . . . I decided to put the boy off, telling him that if he loved me, there was no problem but that he had to wait until the right time.

There were similar findings in the analysis of the results of the nine key informant interviews in Mukono schools. One sixteen-year-old girl reported how she had modeled her sexual avoidance behavior after Sara, especially cautioning girls that going out with sugar daddies would spoil their futures:

I have learnt how to make decisions. I first see what is right and wrong then I act accordingly. I have learnt to think critically before I do something. I have also learnt to advise others, to stop going out with sugar daddies. If not, you land into trouble. I have learnt how I can protect my life. Sara gives me courage to be hard working and get better results. Also, to help others if possible. . . . If I begin going with men at this age, I will get an STD or become pregnant. I want to study hard and be well-off. I want to be a lawyer or a journalist.

In all the interviews, this theme emerged as a major lesson learned by girls. They advised others to avoid discos and blue movies, avoid things they could not afford, and avoid relationships motivated by economic gain. They also commended Sara's role in advising and helping others, such as when she saved her friend Amina who was tricked into drinking alcohol, and was nearly driven off by truck drivers.

A nineteen-year-old girl from Mukono High School first heard about Sara when the lifeskills club started at their school. She reported that in the club, when they talk about Sara, they discuss how to make decisions, create plays, songs, poems, and debates. She stated her reaction toward unwanted sexual advances:

> I was going to market to buy things; then I found a group of teenage boys. They started calling to me. I did not respond. They tried to touch me. They asked me to be their lover. I refused and ran away and went back home. . . . I want to have an education with the aim of getting a job in the future. I do not want to get involved in sex when I am not ready for it. I have three choices: I want to become a journalist, a lawyer, and failing those, I will be a teacher.

The above indicate that girls are influenced by Sara to use various lifeskills to delay sexual debut and to avoid sexual abuse. Girls who were interviewed reported not only being exposed to the Sara stories, but reported discussing these stories, and relating the issues to their own lives. Thus they were developing their lifeskills through critical thinking and self-reflection.

Participants explained that they usually talk about Sara when they meet in their lifeskills clubs. Here they talk about critical thinking, peer resistance, self-esteem, and having the self-awareness to stand up for what you are and do what you think is right for you. They reported being inspired by Sara and applying what they learned to real-life situations. Throughout the interviews, what girls liked most about Sara is her innovative approach to life. For example, in "The Special Gift," after learning about fuel-efficient mud stoves in science class, she made one for her uncle, thereby convincing him that she should not be taken out of school.

In Uganda the Straight Talk Foundation carries out media and school-based programs aimed at behavior development of adolescents through newsmagazines, other print materials, radio programs, and school-based initiatives. Their newsmagazine, *Young Talk*, has incorporated Sara since the mid-1990s. The magazine—which contains a problem page, letters, personal stories, and other features for young adolescents—has a monthly print run of 280,000 copies. Sixteen copies of the English version of *Young Talk* are distributed to each of twelve thousand primary schools in Uganda, where the language of instruction is English.

A survey of 1,380 children in upper primary classes, conducted in 2000, found that 83 percent had read *Young Talk* and that 23 percent of respondents spontaneously recalled Sara from the magazine—double the 1999 recall rate.[25] Sara accounts for 12 to 25 percent of the space in each issue. Teachers were using Sara to build interactive skills:

> We dramatize role plays so that we do not forget the children who are not so comfortable with English. . . . So now we are going to do a role play, playing a man who is drunk, trying to befriend a child.
>
> . . .
>
> [In counseling children] we find most of the time we also refer to some of the things that happen which appear in *Young Talk*. . . . For example, when we are counseling girls, [we discuss] the case of [Sara's friend] Amina.

Teachers need to take a special interest in the Sara material, become familiar with its content, and think about ways it can be used creatively. One teacher from the Mubunga Primary

School, Kisoro, talked about the story "Sara Saves Her Friend": "Children like the story and it is educative. It conveys a message to them because in our locality, this kind of business is common where grown men take these young girls from bars and the girls get problems from there."

The Straight Talk study concluded: (1) Sara continues to be a very popular children's educational comic strip, especially for young adolescents. Sara characters were spontaneously identified by at least one out of four of the youngest children surveyed. (2) Children and adults can both appreciate the educational qualities of the Sara animated cartoon and can successfully use it in different learning settings. (3) Sara cartoons are effective communication tools, even with children with low English proficiency. (4) Sara is used in a variety of ways to guide children through interactive learning methods, including discussions and role plays. (5) Teachers and children both find that Sara portrays characters who are like themselves. The Sara materials directly speak to the children about friendships, relationships, and problem solving.[26]

Sustaining Sara as a Brand

Mid-term evaluation suggested that UNICEF should capitalize on the Sara investment and expand the SCI in other countries of sub-Saharan Africa. In some countries there is good evidence that various organizations are beginning to use Sara materials. When Sara was conceived, it was recognized that the Sara products would have a potential to be marketed beyond UNICEF, and that the SCI should be made into a self-sustaining enterprise.[27] Beginning in 1996 a search was undertaken for a regional publisher that would have the capacity to market, distribute, and sell Sara products throughout the sub-Sahara. Ultimately, a copublishing and marketing agreement was signed between UNICEF and Maskew Miller Longman (MML), South Africa, a regional educational publisher with a wide reach throughout Africa. Sara materials for readers and teachers are being developed by MML for broad distribution in educational systems across Africa. Plans have been discussed to fully exploit the Sara "brand" through the development of Sara products, including school accessories, clothes, and dishware.

Very often communication programs die quickly with no trace, except perhaps in libraries and repositories. Sara is now being adopted by other program implementation and donor groups because Sara products are available through a commercial channel. This bodes well for the growth and sustainability of the SCI, and UNICEF is discussing the feasibility of housing Sara in a foundation, or an NGO, to complement the commercial initiative. These moves toward sustainability make the SCI a unique project in development communication.

Sara has the potential to be recognized widely throughout sub-Saharan Africa as a symbol for girls' empowerment in the face of HIV/AIDS. Where a reasonable attempt has been made to carry out good programs with Sara stories and tools, Sara becomes a supportive, positive role model for girls. However, to be realistic, a communication initiative cannot solve the HIV/AIDS pandemic by itself. It must be designed to support changes in the overall environment, such as access to youth-friendly and high-quality health and educational services.

The SCI has demonstrated that engaging cartoon characters, when well researched and programmed, can engender discussion in communities and help shift individual behaviors and community norms. Sara is being adopted by many user groups in the fight against HIV/AIDS in Africa. Her added value is that she appeals to all age groups and triggers discussion between generations. The SCI's promise lies in that it represents a set of communication tools that have a wide research base and are applicable across many cultures. The commercialization of Sara materials through an educational publisher (and potentially a foundation or NGO) bodes well for future sustainability. Sara stands side-by-side with African girls to address the inequality they face by virtue of their gender.

Notes

1. S. Bader and H. Wach, "Gender HIV/AIDS Transmission and Impacts: A Review of Issues and Evidence," Report of the Swedish International Development Cooperation Agency (SIDA), Stockholm, 1998; Lynellyn D. Long and E. Maxine Ankrah, eds., *Women's Experience with HIV/AIDS* (New York: Columbia University Press, 1996).

2. S. Watstein and R. Laurich, *AIDS and Women: A Source Book* (Phoenix: Oryx Press, 1991), 159.

3. Recent data is beginning to show that uncircumcised males are at equal or more risk than females. See D. D. Halberin and R. C. Bailey, "Male Circumcision and HIV Infection: Ten Years and Counting," *Lancet* 354 (1999): 1813–15.

4. W. Mbugua, "Gender and HIV/AIDS: Social Mobilization and the Role of Leaders," Report of the UNFPA-Organized Breakout Panel, Africa Development Forum, Addis Ababa, December 2000.

5. Rachel Carnegie and Rhona Birrell Weisen, "The Ability to Act: Strengthening People's Lifeskills," in *Involving People, Evolving Behaviour*, ed. N. McKee et al., (Penang: Southbound/UNICEF, 2000): 121–54.

6. A. K. Blanc, "The Effect of Power in Sexual Relationships on Reproductive and Sexual Health: An Examination of the Evidence," paper prepared for the Population Council for discussion at the Meeting on Power in Sexual Relationships, Washington, D.C., March 1–2, 2001.

7. Neill McKee, "The Adolescent Girl Communication Initiative of Eastern and Southern Africa," in *Drawing Insight: Communicating Development through Animation*, ed. J. Greene and D. Reber (Penang: Southbound/UNICEF, 1996), 50–54.

8. Patrick Coleman and Rita Meyer, eds., "Entertainment for Social Change," Enter-Educate Conference, Johns Hopkins University Center for Communication Programs, Baltimore, March 29–April 1, 1989.

9. George McBean and Neill McKee, "The Animated Film in Development Communication," in *Drawing Insight: Communicating Development through Animation*, ed. J. Greene and D. Reber (Penang: Southbound/UNICEF, 1996), 10–15.

10. Rachel Carnegie, *Meeting Meena: Documentation Study on Utilisation of Meena Communication Initiative*, (Kathmandu: UNICEF Regional Office for South Asia, 2001).

11. Neill McKee, Erma Manoncourt, Chin Saik Yoon, and Rachel Carnegie, eds., *Involving People, Evolving Behaviour* (Penang: Southbound/UNICEF, 2000).

12. Carnegie and Birrell Weisen, "Ability to Act," 121–54.

13. "Facing the Challenges of HIV/AIDS/STDs: A Gender-Based Response," report of the Royal Tropical Institute, Amsterdam, and Southern Africa AIDS Information Dissemination Service, Harare, 1998.

14. UNAIDS/WHO, "Report on the global HIV/AIDS epidemic," (Geneva: Joint United Nations Programme on HIV/AIDS and World Health Organization, June 2000).

15. T. Barton, *Epidemic and Behaviours: A Review of Changes in Ugandan Sexual Behaviour in the Early 1990s* (Kampala: UNAIDS, January 1997); E. C. Green, "The Impact of Religious Organizations in Promoting HIV/AIDS Prevention," revised version of paper presented at Challenges for the Church: AIDS, Malaria and TB, Christian Connections for International Health, Arlington, Va., May 25–26, 2001.

16. UNICEF, "Formative Research Process in the Sara Communication Initiative: A Report and Resource Book, Eastern and Southern Africa Regional Office," UNICEF Regional Office for Eastern and Southern Africa, Nairobi, Sept 1999.

17. Mira Aghi, "Formative Research in the Meena Communication Initiative," in *Drawing Insight: Communicating Development through Animation*, ed. J. Greene and D. Reber (Penang: Southbound/ UNICEF, 1996), 37–43.

18. UNICEF, "Formative Research Process."

19. C. Russon, "Evaluation of the Sara Communication Initiative:

Final Summary," Evaluation Center, Western Michigan University, November 2000.

20. Ibid.

21. M. C. Y. Mbago and F. J. Sichona, "Sara Communication Initiative Outcomes Study in Tanzania," Demographic Training Unit, University of Dar-es-Salaam, November 1999.

22. P. Alila and M. Omasa, "Qualitative Outcome Study: The Sara Communication Initiative," Institute of Development Studies, College of Humanities and Social Sciences, University of Nairobi, 2000.

23. A. Nuwagaba and S. Neema, "Evaluation of Sara Communication Initiative: The Case of FAWE Schools," Makerere Institute of Social Research, Makerere University, Kampala, July 2000.

24. FAWE, "Programme Operations Document," Forum for African Women Educationists, Uganda Chapter, Kampala, July 2000.

25. Lillian Mutengu, Patrick Walugembe, and Susan Kasedde, "*Sara* Representations," *Young Talk* Evaluation Report, Straight Talk Foundation, Kampala, November 2000.

26. Ibid.

27. McKee, "Adolescent Girl Communication."

12

The Treatment of AIDS in *Soul Buddyz*

A Multimedia Campaign for Children's Health in South Africa

*Sue Goldstein, Shereen Usdin, Esca Scheepers,
Aadielah Anderson, and Garth Japhet*

South Africa has more people living with HIV/AIDS than any other country in the world. An estimated 4.7 million people there are infected with the HIV virus.[1] While the country has a reasonable GDP per capita ($6,900 in 1999),[2] the distribution of wealth is skewed. Many people live below the poverty line.[3] The apartheid system caused huge social dislocation, tearing families apart and making migration a way of life.[4] The education system for black South Africans was downgraded and systematically undermined.[5] While the present South African constitution promotes equality, women are disempowered. Women and children face the highest levels of poverty, and the level of violence against women is very high.[6]

Compared to most of the continent, the reach of media in South Africa is particularly good: television reaches about three-quarters of the population, radio reaches over 90 percent, and newspapers reach 40 percent.[7] According to UNICEF, there are 316 radio sets and 118 TV sets for every thousand people.[8]

The population of South Africa is young. Some 40 percent of South Africans are under eighteen; there are about 13 million children between five and eighteen.[9] Each year a large cohort of young, vulnerable South Africans becomes sexually active. As most of the AIDS deaths occur among people twenty to fifty years old, many children have parents, siblings, and relatives who either are HIV positive, are sick and need care, or have died.[10] By 2005 one million South African children will be AIDS orphans.[11] *Soul Buddyz* uses a multimedia intervention to motivate and mobilize communities to support the health and social needs of South Africa's children.[12]

From *Soul City* to *Soul Buddyz*

Entertainment-education (edutainment) is seen internationally as a powerful educational tool.[13] The power of edutainment rests in its ability to model positive attitudes and behaviors through characters with whom the audience bonds. The characters come to play an integral part in the lives of the audience members, who experience life lessons vicariously.[14] Also, many educational media programs are unable to attract large audiences; entertainment-education integrates educational issues into entertaining formats, enabling health promoters to secure prime-time mass-media slots. In some instances, the ability to attract advertising revenue or local sponsorship allows for partnerships of mutual benefit to develop between broadcasters and health promoters.

The Soul City Institute for Health and Development Communication is an NGO established in South Africa in 1992 to address a wide range of health and development issues through television and radio dramas, newspaper inserts, advertising and marketing, and media advocacy. *Soul City* has become a household name in South Africa. Independent evaluations have shown its ability to have an impact on a variety of health issues by conveying information, by increasing debate and interpersonal interaction, and by changing attitudes, practices, and social norms.[15] The television series alone reaches more than 17 million South Africans and has been broadcast in a number of other African countries, including Zambia, Botswana, and Namibia.[16]

Soul City uses the five pillars of the Ottawa Charter for Health Promotion to help define the scope and context of its communication interventions: (1) promoting healthy public policy, (2) creating supportive environments, (3) supporting community action for health, (4) developing personal skills, and (5) reorienting health services.[17] The key aspects of the Soul City methodology are illustrated in figure 12.1.

Through a thorough formative research process, health and development messages about such topics as HIV/AIDS, youth sexuality, and domestic violence are designed and integrated into the edutainment vehicle (see fig. 12.2). Care is taken to

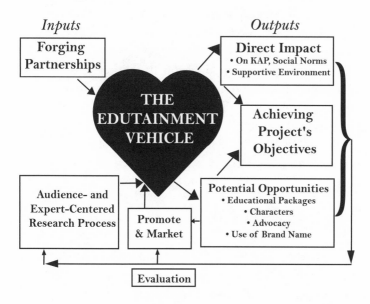

Fig. 12.1. The Soul City edutainment model

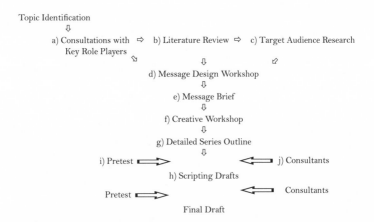

Fig. 12.2. The formative research process

ensure that the media materials are of the highest quality. The television and radio dramas portray realistic situations so that audiences can identify with the characters, and the stories are highly emotional in order to not only impart knowledge but change attitudes.

Soul City is extremely popular with children under sixteen, even though the materials were designed for youth and adults. In the light of this, coupled with the seriousness of the AIDS epidemic and the importance of intervening at an early age, the Soul City Institute created a second edutainment series, *Soul Buddyz*, for children between eight and twelve.

Designing and Implementing *Soul Buddyz*

The development process for *Soul Buddyz* was similar to the process followed for the *Soul City* series, except that pilot episodes of the *Soul Buddyz* television and radio series and print materials were produced before the campaign was fully developed. The testing of the pilot materials with parents, teachers, child care workers, and children across the nine provinces of South Africa helped shape the *Soul Buddyz* vehicle. For example, the radio pilot, produced by a well-respected company, used adults to portray children's voices instead of working with child actors. This alerted the Soul City Institute to the fact that there were no radio programs in South Africa for eight- to twelve-year-old children and that radio producers had little experience working with children and no experience in producing children's drama. With help from the BBC, the *Soul Buddyz* project subsequently organized a program to train South African radio producers to work with children. Further, the pilot testing showed that adults needed assistance in parenting skills, especially in communicating with children and how to sensitively handle discipline. The development of the *Soul Buddyz* parenting booklet was a direct outcome of the pilot process.

The *Soul Buddyz* materials were developed in partnership with the educational branch of the broadcaster, SABC Educational Television; with a number of NGOs (such as Drive Alive, the National Association of People Living with AIDS, and the National Council of Child and Family Welfare); and with children. NGO services such as the toll-free Childline were often integrated into the *Soul Buddyz* storyline. For example, the plot about sexual abuse showed a child learning how to use the Childline, which provides counseling and follow-up services to children. The Childline phone number was prominently displayed after each *Soul Buddyz* episode as well as in all print materials.

The Messages of *Soul* Buddyz

The AIDS-related messages in *Soul Buddyz* were both general and specific. The general messages related to self-esteem and gender:

- I am unique and have my own strengths and weaknesses—
we are all different and special in our own way. All people
deserve respect irrespective of age, gender, religion, race,
or state of health or impairment. They have strengths
and weaknesses just like you and me.

This message underpinned the entire *Soul Buddyz* series and
was continuously conveyed through the composition of the "Soul
Buddyz" group, whose members were from different racial and
socioeconomic backgrounds and had different abilities. Formative research for the series showed that children who were different in any way were teased and bullied by others.

- It is important to serve the community to which I belong
and to recognize that my actions or lack of action influence and affect others.

This message called for community action around the various educational issues, including AIDS, and promoted the idea
of peer-based support. The storyline for the entire series was
a competition for which each group of children had to do three
community projects and were then visited by a judge who discussed the projects with them. The series culminated in an
international children's rights convention, at which the prize
was awarded.

- Boys and girls are equal and deserve equal respect. Girls
can do anything—though it may sometimes be difficult.
Boys are allowed to "feel" and be sensitive.

Formative research showed that girls in South Africa felt
anxious about the strong possibility of being abused. A few
episodes were dedicated to this message; they showed girls as-
piring to things, like becoming a pilot, that many South African children believe are not possible. Great care was taken
throughout the series not to stereotype gender roles.

- I need to identify my feelings and learn to express them in an appropriate way. Children have the right to dream and hope and to the space to articulate those dreams and hopes. Children have the right to be worried and have concerns and should be encouraged to express these worries so that they may be addressed.

Formative research showed that children did not know how to express their emotions. Telling each story from the perspective of a child, and in such a way that the audience could hear the child's inner dialogue through a voice-over technique, allowed children to understand, in words, what a character was feeling and thus how to express emotions.

- Life is about choices. It is important to realize that your choices will influence your future and can affect others.

A problem-solving approach was encouraged, and children were shown looking for their own answers and trying different solutions. Children were encouraged to take responsibility for their actions.

More specific statements treat issues about AIDS and sexuality:

- It is important to communicate about AIDS and sex. It is often difficult to get information about sensitive issues but it's important to keep on trying to get accurate information. Friends and adults are not always right, so cross-check your information with other sources.

Before the series most children had heard about AIDS, though their knowledge was sketchy. They knew that AIDS was incurable, but believed it involved getting sores and going mad. Neither the invisible nature of HIV infection nor its methods of transmission were clearly understood: "If you stand next to them they infect you. If they have it, then you'll also get it," said a ten-year-old boy. Formative research also showed that parents found it very difficult to talk about sex with their children.[18] One story, covering several episodes, is about a young boy who learns that his mother has AIDS; he then goes through a process of learning the facts about AIDS in a few different ways, and one of the ways (from a school friend) proves to be inaccurate.

- My body is my own. It is normal to feel uncomfortable with changes which happen to one's body at the time of puberty. Children have the right to say no to sex and abuse.

One story shows a romance between two young teens. The girl is experiencing menarche and finding out about puberty; at the same time the young boy has a wet dream and has all the myths surrounding this dispelled. In another story a young girl who has been sexually abused by her uncle is assisted by the Childline and one of her friends to get adult help.

Soul Buddyz as a Multimedia Edutainment Vehicle

The *Soul Buddyz* multimedia vehicle consists of a television drama series, a radio magazine show, lifeskills print materials for children, and a parenting booklet. The twenty-six-episode television series revolves around the lives of eight child characters (the Soul Buddyz) who handle issues such as starting at a new school, being bullied, and having a mother who has AIDS—issues that confront South African children in their everyday lives (fig. 12.3). The Soul Buddyz are of mixed race, socioeconomic class, and gender (fig. 12.4). At the end of each episode, a dozen children from all over South Africa are shown commenting on the educational issues raised. Each episode unfolds from the perspective of one of the Soul Buddyz, whose inner thoughts are conveyed by a voice-over. Each episode also includes a fantasy sequence to illustrate the hopes and fears of

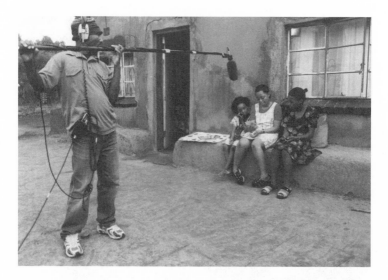

Fig. 12.3. Filming an episode of the South African television series *Soul Buddyz* in which Karabo (center) and Ndhivuo (right), two of the series' four Soul Buddyz, take care of their friend's sister, Sihle (left). Sihle's mother died of AIDS, and her father is very ill. Soul City Institute of Health and Development Communication. Used with permission.

children. A rap song in each episode emphasizes the main educational message. The series is multilingual. The main language of each episode is English, but each child uses his or her own language (subtitled in English) when at home, when talking with parents or siblings, or when using the voice-over technique.

The radio component consisted of a twenty-six-episode radio magazine, also called *Soul Buddyz*. The thirty-minute magazine incorporated a radio drama with child protagonists, a dramatized information segment for adults and children, and a phone-in talk show with young presenters and expert guests (fig. 12.5). The program was broadcast in three South African languages (Setswana, North Sotho, Xhosa) to appeal to a wide audience.

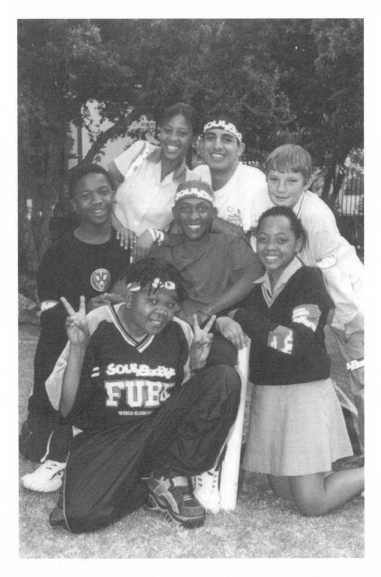

Fig. 12.4. The main cast of *Soul Buddyz*. Soul City Institute of Health and Development Communication. Used with permission.

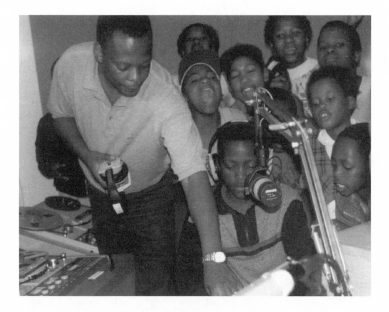

Fig. 12.5. A studio-based training program for children involved in recording the *Soul Buddyz* radio drama. Soul City Institute of Health and Development Communication. Used with permission.

A vibrant lifeskills book was distributed to a million seventh-grade students in every primary school in South Africa. The interactive lifeskills book, illustrated with photos of the Soul Buddyz, cover all the topics treated in the television series in an abbreviated comic strip format. Also included are true-life stories as told by children (who remain anonymous), activities for children, and educators' notes.

A user-friendly parenting booklet was distributed through the *Sunday Times* (whose circulation of six hundred thousand is the nation's largest) and various South African NGOs. Although the literacy rate in South Africa is relatively high—82 percent of adults (those over fifteen) are literate—the average reading level is not very high. The parenting booklet was produced in three languages (English, Afrikaans, and Zulu) at the fifth-grade level. The booklet covers topics such as communication, discipline, resolving conflicts, single parenting, building children's self-esteem, and preventing child accidents. It also describes ways to talk to children about sexuality, HIV/AIDS, and death.

Because of the low levels of sexual literacy among South African children, a six-minute animated sex-education video was produced for the television series. The animation helped overcome the problem of showing sexual organs on national television and facilitated an open discussion on the topic. In an episode in which the Soul Buddyz are confused about sex, a friendly nurse sits them down and shows them the video. This was the first time such explicit material had been televised in South Africa. To maximize the usefulness of the video, the episode was condensed to a popular twelve-minute tape sold to schools and parents as a teaching aid.

The Soul Buddyz project also included an advocacy component with five AIDS-related focal areas: (1) using the news media, (2) training NGOs to engage the news media, (3) creating resource booklets for journalists on children's rights and HIV/AIDS, (4) training journalists in children's rights, and (5) launching a campaign to secure social security rights for all children, including those infected and affected by HIV/AIDS.

The Impact of *Soul Buddyz*

An evaluation of *Soul Buddyz* was commissioned in early 2001 to gauge the audience reach and reception of *Soul Buddyz* and to investigate its impact. A nationwide survey of two thousand individuals as well as qualitative interviews (nine focus group and eighteen in-depth) were conducted among children aged eight to thirteen. Some fifteen hundred survey interviews, six focus group interviews, and eighteen in-depth interviews were conducted among parents and caregivers (of the randomly selected school children). Fifty structured interviews and six semistructured interviews were conducted with, respectively, school principals and teachers.

After its first season of television and radio broadcasts, three-quarters of all respondents aged eight to thirteen had heard of *Soul Buddyz,* and two-thirds reported that they had watched, listened to, or used the Soul Buddyz materials. The television series also reached over a third of parents or adult caregivers. Almost half the children who watched *Soul Buddyz* on television (on the country's most popular audience channel, SABC 1) reported that they watched "all or most of the episodes." And even though not all rural radio stations were used, the Soul Buddyz materials (television series, radio magazine, booklets) reached a remarkable 41 percent of the rural children.

Both quantitative and qualitative analyses indicated that Soul Buddyz media materials were highly relevant to their primary target audience;[19] many found them enjoyable and educational. In addition to the children, parents, caregivers, and teachers were all highly supportive of *Soul Buddyz.* As one parent said, "*Soul Buddyz* is a bonus. It deals with real-life issues and real-life situations and makes them [children] more aware of things which are a reality."

Impact on Gender, Youth Sexuality, and HIV / AIDS

Soul Buddyz consistently affected the quality and frequency of discussion of issues among audience members. More than three-quarters of the children who watched the television series said they talked about the things they saw with other people. And parents and other caregivers who watched *Soul Buddyz* were more likely to discuss issues of sexuality with their children, compared to parents who had not watched. A rural parent noted, "I like that *Soul Buddyz* teaches kids things that are not easy for parents to talk to their kids about."

Children exposed to Soul Buddyz media materials were more likely to discuss HIV/AIDS than were children who were not exposed. Three-quarters of eleven- to thirteen-year-olds with high exposure to the television series reported talking about HIV/AIDS (compared to 61 percent of same-age respondents who were not exposed). One young viewer noted, "It [*Soul Buddyz*] has changed the way I interact with my friends, parents, and people in the community; I have learnt to be more respectful, and I have learnt to talk about things that are of great concern to me or that hurt me."

Exposure to *Soul Buddyz* was associated with increased knowledge as well as positive attitudes on a number of youth sexuality issues. For instance, two-thirds of the boys with high exposure to the television series disagreed with the statement, "A person has to have sex with their boyfriend or girlfriend to show they love them." Children exposed to the *Soul Buddyz* television series were more likely to agree with the statement "boys and girls are equal."

Exposure to any of the three *Soul Buddyz* media components (television, radio, booklets) was positively associated with knowledge about HIV/AIDS and with the frequency that condom use was mentioned as a way of preventing contracting HIV/AIDS. Children exposed to *Soul Buddyz* on television were more likely to know that people with HIV can look healthy, and children exposed to any of the three Soul Buddyz media components were more likely than children with no exposure to mention consistent condom use as a way of preventing HIV/AIDS.

Qualitative data showed that *Soul Buddyz* messages about care and support for people living with HIV/AIDS came across clearly and effectively. One young child said, "*Soul Buddyz* teaches me about AIDS. Like when one of the boys' mother had AIDS, it shows how a person can cope with AIDS." *Soul Buddyz* also seemed to play an important role in addressing the stigma of HIV/AIDS. Children exposed to the television series were more likely to say that they were willing to be friends with someone who has HIV/AIDS.

Lessons Learned

The Soul Buddyz experience demonstrates that it is possible to use an edutainment strategy to reach and teach children about difficult topics. Evaluation of the program suggests the following reasons for its power:

- *Soul Buddyz* increased children's knowledge about gender, sexuality, and AIDS and enhanced their problem-solving and communication skills with peers and adults.
- At the level of community action or social mobilization, many of our children respondents reported forming support groups (reflecting the *Soul Buddyz* storyline). The Soul Buddyz support group in the television series undoubtedly inspired some of them.
- Adults who watched *Soul Buddyz* increasingly realized that children have rights and can contribute to building a better society. Further, *Soul Buddyz* helped them to communicate more effectively with children about sexuality and other sensitive topics.
- Nearly all teachers (94 percent) felt that *Soul Buddyz* had given them a new understanding of the problems faced by children.

Production Challenges

The production of both broadcast series faced several challenges. Not only was there virtually no prior experience in South Africa of producing children's radio drama, the commercialization of the state media had relegated children's programming to the back burner. However, the pilot of *Soul Buddyz* radio magazine on the three radio stations was very successful, and other stations were inspired to participate. And stations were pleased with the audience response to the phone-in sections of the radio magazine. Lessons were learned about the appropriate airing times for this type of program (for instance, when children are in not school), and that both adults and children appreciate such programs. As a result of the effectiveness of the first set of *Soul Buddyz* broadcasts (in three languages), in July 2003 all nine African-language stations plan to air the second *Soul Buddyz* series.

The broadcast of the *Soul Buddyz* television program in multiple languages (with English subtitles) worked well with audience members, and even the younger children had no difficulty understanding the content. The use of multiple languages is particularly important in a multicultural society in which English is increasingly becoming dominant and children's home languages are being eroded. The television series was carefully crafted to be as visual as possible so that children could understand the stories and messages without understanding each word.

In any effective mass media intervention, full participation of audience members is essential. In the Soul Buddyz project, children participated in various ways: from developing the campaign logo and slogan, to detailed interaction with the scripts, to the writing of the rap songs. Children suggested several of the storylines. One innovative aspect of including their participation was to show children the twenty-six episodes prior to airing so they could comment on each episode in their own language. These comments were broadcast at the end of each episode as "Buddyz Buzz."

Soul Buddyz has begun to make a contribution to the health and development process of South African children. The program has demonstrated that through edutainment in the mass media serious issues like HIV/AIDS can be dealt with effectively and that the message can be fun and extremely popular. Children in South Africa, irrespective of their race or language, learned a great deal from this intervention, and it clearly is shaping their attitudes and intended behaviors for the future. Shaping the attitudes of future teenagers—and their parents—will be critical in shaping the future of the AIDS epidemic and thus of the entire country.

Notes

1. UNAIDS/WHO, *AIDS Epidemic Update, December 2001;* UNAIDS, <http://www.unaids.org/worldaidsday/2001/Epiupdate 2001/Epiupdate2001_en.pdf>, 2002.

2. Winthrop Corporation, *Corporate Information for South Africa,* <www.corporateinformation.com/zacorp.html>, 2000.

3. Michael Samson, Oliver Babson, Claudia Haarman, Dirk Haarman, Gilbert Khathi, Kenneth Mac Quene, and Ingrid van Niekerk, *Research Review on Social Security Reform and the Basic Income Grant for South Africa* (Cape Town: Economic Policy Research Institute, 2002).

4. Nicoli Nattrass, *Growth, Employment, and Economic Policy in South Africa: A Critical Review,* <www.cde.org.za/pub_cde-focus. html>, 1998.

5. Shireen Motala, Helen Perry, John Aitchison, Jane Castle, and Tamar Ruth, *Quarterly Review of Education and Training in South Africa* 8 (2001): 16–21.

6. South African Police Services, *The Reported Serious Crime Situation in South Africa for the Period January–September 2001,* <www. saps.org.za/8_crimeinfo/200112/report.htm>, 2001.

7. South African Advertising Research Foundation, *Living Standards Measures* (Johannesburg: SAARF, 1999).

8. UNICEF, *The State of the World's Children 2000* (New York: Oxford University Press, 2000).

9. UNICEF, *The State of the World's Children 1998* (New York: Oxford University Press, 1998).

10. Rose Smart, *Children Living with HIV/AIDS in South Africa: A Rapid Appraisal* (Johannesburg: Save the Children/Interim National HIV/AIDS Care and Support Task Team, 2000).

11. Department of Health, *HIV/AIDS Strategic Plan for South Africa, 2000–2005* (Pretoria: Department of Health, 2000).

12. *Soul Buddyz* is seen as an extension of the Soul City vehicle, but specially designed for children. The word *Soul* in the title, and in the same font, is the brand link between the two; the intention was to recruit audiences as early as possible, as children would recognize the link.

13. D. Lawrence Kincaid, Sung Hee Yun, Phyllis T. Poitrow, and Yasar Yaser, "Turkey's Mass Media Family Planning Campaign," in *Organizational Aspects of Health Communication Campaigns*, ed. T. E. Backer and E. M. Rogers (Newbury Park, Calif.: Sage, 1993), 68.

14. Arvind Singhal and Everett M. Rogers, *Entertainment-Education, A Communication Strategy for Social Change* (Mahwah, N.J.: Lawrence Erlbaum Associates, 1999).

15. This phenomenon is known as parasocial interaction. M. J. Papa, A. Singhal, S. Law, S. Pant, S. Sood, E. M. Rogers, and C. L. Shefner-Rogers, "Entertainment-Education and Social Change: An Analysis of Parasocial Interaction, Social Learning, Collective Efficiency, and Paradoxical Communication," *Journal of Communication* 50, 4 (2000): 31–55.

16. Esca Scheepers, *Soul City 4 Evaluation Results—Integrated Summary Report, 2001* (Johannesburg: Institute for Health and Development Communication), <http://www.soulcity.org.za/>.

17. WHO, Ottawa Charter. (Geneva: World Health Organization, 2002), <http://www.who.int/hpr/archive/docs/ottawa.html>.

18. In a national survey in South Africa, only 14 percent of twelve- to seventeen-year-olds said that they learned about sex from their parents.

19. Relevance was assessed through items like the following: "*Soul Buddyz* helps me with things that happen in my life" (true/false) and "Is there anything in *Soul Buddyz* that reminds you of your own life?" (open-ended response), and through analysis of open-ended items around likes, dislikes, and what respondents had learned from *Soul Buddyz*. Relevance was qualitatively assessed through respondents' spontaneous remarks and assessment of *Soul Buddyz*.

13

"HIV Is Gold, AIDS Is Platinum"

Community Radio for Social Change

Tanja Bosch

High school youth crowd into the auditorium of Princeton High School in Cape Town dancing enthusiastically to the sounds of their favorite hip-hop groups—Prophets of the City, Brasse Vannie Kaap, and Devious. This is not an unusual sight in Cape Town, where hip-hop music is very popular among the youth. But listen carefully and you'll hear that these lyrics are unconventional—they deal with sexuality, HIV, and AIDS, alerting youth to prevention issues and advising them how to conduct their relationships. The concert, hosted by local community radio station Bush Radio, marks World AIDS Day, December 1, 2000. Between hip-hop mixes a spontaneous break-dance performance erupts on the dance floor, while the Bush Radio DJs engage the audience with issues of HIV/AIDS.

This concert formed part of a Bush Radio campaign aimed at educating youth in Cape Town's townships about HIV/AIDS. As the AIDS pandemic sweeps across Africa, strategies to effect behavior change are constantly being reinvented. The more creative of these—like Bush Radio's hip-hop campaign Youth against AIDS 2000—transcend traditional approaches,

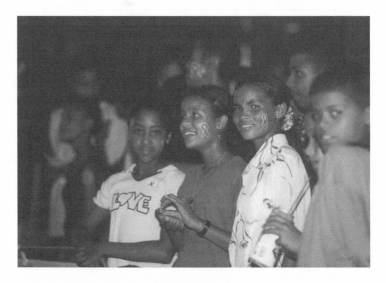

Fig. 13.1. Youths celebrate World AIDS Day (2000) at the Bush Radio hip-hop concert in Cape Town. Bush Radio. Photograph by Juanita Williams. Used with permission.

deliberately mixing entertaining formats with messages for social change.[1]

Bush Radio in Postapartheid South Africa

The transformation of legal and constitutional contexts in postapartheid South Africa, particularly the creation of a new constitution, allowed for freedom of expression and guaranteed media protection through the Bill of Rights.[2] The Independent Broadcast Authority (IBA) was set up by the government in 1994 to democratize the airwaves, to protect broadcasts from government interference, and to encourage ownership and control of broadcasts by previously disadvantaged groups.[3] The IBA granted eighty-two community licenses and various commercial licenses and also started opening up the television airwaves.

Bush Radio, perhaps the oldest community radio project in the country, was one of the stations granted a community broadcast license. It began as a cassette education project of the Talking Newspaper Pilot Project (TNPP) in February 1988. The TNPP masked a broader political agenda in the articulation of its goals. It was established to provide access to the print media for illiterate and blind people, as part of the University of Cape Town's Community Adult Education Program. Listener feedback prompted an improvement in programming, and with growing support from progressive organizations an audiocassette service organization, the Cassette Education Project (CASET), was set up in 1989.[4] CASET produced cassette recordings of conferences and political meetings, local music, poetry, and storytelling. CASET proposed a community radio network to community organizations in Cape Town in March 1991, resulting in a series of monthly open forums in the name of Bush Radio.[5]

The Context of Hip-Hop in South Africa

Music has always played a central role in the political and cultural life of South Africa. Musicians, artists, and playwrights were key in acquiring support against the oppressive apartheid regime.[6] Music for black South Africans—from Afro-jazz to *isicathamiya* (choral music)—functioned much like blues music for blacks during and after slavery in the United States: it sustained them during apartheid, enabling them to maintain their humanity and acting as a kind of healing force.[7]

Hip-hop emerged on the Cape Flats in the early 1980s as one of many responses to apartheid. Particularly powerful in Cape Town, hip-hop channeled the tensions of being racially marginalized from local domains of power.[8] It is still popular among youth in Cape Town, who use the music in the construction of their ethnic identities. Local hip-hop musicians have a large following in Cape Town's townships, and use their music in stimulating community development initiatives.

The Youth against AIDS Campaign

Bush Radio launched its AIDS-education campaign, Youth against AIDS (YAA) 2000, in March 2000, utilizing the power of radio, hip-hop, and live performance. The campaign was supported through funding from the Dutch Institute for Southern Africa and the Madunia Foundation of the Netherlands. YAA 2000 took place within the broader framework of the South African Community Radio AIDS Initiative, which involved seven stations in the National Community Radio Forum.

The main aim of the campaign was to produce effective ways to educate high school youth, especially in Bush Radio's broadcast area, on issues of sexuality and AIDS: "YAA 2000 is more than just a fun live event under the AIDS banner, it is a creative platform of performance and participation, which aims to build a new level of awareness around AIDS and sexuality in Cape Town townships, and particularly among the youth."[9]

South Africa is said to have the most people infected with HIV/AIDS on the continent, and a provincial survey on HIV/AIDS shows that HIV is on the rise among teenagers in the Western Cape, with increasing numbers of pregnant teenagers testing positive.[10] Bush Radio producer Shaheen Ariefdien passionately argues, "Although hip-hop has been incorporated into mass culture to some extent . . . hip-hop is political." Ariefdien explained that because hip-hop is perceived by youth as antiestablishment, and thus is considered credible, it has the potential to reach youth.

Before launching the YAA campaign, a Bush Radio research team assessed the knowledge and attitudes of the targeted youth, then incorporated the results into the format and themes of the radio programs. Ariefdien explains that stigmatization, misconceptions, and conspiracy theories (about the origin of the HIV virus) were the most common themes. For example, a common explanation of the acronym AIDS is American Ideology to Discourage Sex. A song by a local artist, "Conspiracy Theories," argues that whatever the cause of AIDS, controlling it is the important issue. Another important aim of the YAA campaign was the building of local capacity through the experience gained from formative research, as well as the organization of other campaign activities.

The campaign included live performances and a simultaneous live radio broadcast from Princeton High in Mitchell's Plain, one of Cape Town's largest townships. The station produced a CD of the event with the aim of encouraging youth ownership and raising the campaign's profile. Bush Radio and Radio Netherlands distributed the CD (at no cost) to community radio stations, nationally and internationally.

Another aspect of the YAA campaign was weekly township school lunchtime shows, held at Princeton High School. The meetings were designed in consultation with local high schools, their students, members of the Representative Council of Learners, and Bush Radio's Youth Outreach workers. The Bush Radio crew brought their equipment to Princeton High every month, inviting all students, including those from neighboring high schools, to come and chat about sexuality.

During the lunchtime shows, students found it difficult to engage in discussions openly with teachers and parents present. This led to a series of after-school meetings. Rap lyrics would blast out in a local auditorium, and in the relaxed atmosphere

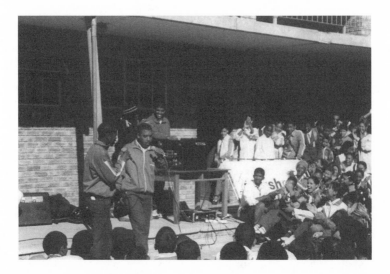

Fig. 13.2. DJs from Bush Radio conduct HIV education at a school in Cape Town. Bush Radio. Photograph by Juanita Williams. Used with permission.

teenagers frankly stated their views on sex and asked questions about AIDS. The explosive lyrics of local and international songs hung in the air: "Conspiracy Theories," "Ins and Outs," and "HIV Is Gold, AIDS Is Platinum" (with its reference to the Grammy Awards).

Bush Radio hoped that its Teen Town Meetings would contribute to the demystification of community radio and the development of youth programming, as it was engaging youth to openly discuss matters of sex and HIV/AIDS. Bush Radio visited over fifteen township schools, showing how radio can highlight youth's challenges and problems. Guest speakers included local doctors and representatives of the Departments of Health and Education. At one meeting HIV testing was made available to students in the auditorium. The youths talked about everything—from nonpenetrative sex, to the male ego, to a young woman's self-esteem when pressured into sex.[11]

Following the broadcasts, Princeton High faculty officially endorsed their students' participation in a daily on-air afternoon radio program, during an intensive one-week campaign. These programs, which involved panels of AIDS experts, school representatives, and youth, tackled attitudes, sexuality, and the prevention, care, and management of HIV/AIDS. The on-air component of the YAA campaign, HIV-Hop Radio, was a five-week radio campaign launched on May 9, 2000. The HIV-Hop show served as a pilot project in the development of a new radio format for youth education. The show was designed after conducting focus group interviews with students from schools in three of the main target communities: Mitchell's Plain, Gugulethu, and Woodstock. The HIV-Hop show was modeled on the station's already highly successful Friday night hip-hop show, hosted by musicians from the community. HIV-Hop segments were rebroadcast during the Friday night program. In both instances listeners called in and engaged in animated on-air discussions.

A key aspect of the youth AIDS campaign was the enthusiastic support of local hip-hop musicians. These celebrity musicians participated in concerts, community events, and on radio shows. They attended workshops with experts to improve their knowledge of HIV/AIDS so they could provide informed inputs during the broadcasts and incorporate social messages into their lyrics.

With so many people both infected and at risk from HIV/AIDS in South Africa, it has become essential to find entertaining and relevant ways to reach youth. Community radio can play a crucial role in targeting this vulnerable population. With its relative independence from advertisers, proximity to the community it serves, and ability to implement locally relevant programs, community radio has a distinct niche in confronting AIDS. As producer Ariefdien points out, "we do whatever we need to do . . . we don't have to play the Top Ten or whatever, but we go into the high schools, and we go outside and broadcast on the pavement if necessary!"

Two years after its launch in 2000, the Bush Radio entertainment-education strategy continues with HIV-Hop segments on its Saturday afternoon youth program and with hip-hop music continually used to engage youth in discussions on globalization, politics, and public health.

Notes

1. A. Singhal and E. Rogers, *Entertainment-Education: A Communication Strategy for Social Change* (Mahwah, N.J.: Lawrence Erlbaum Associates, 1999).

2. S. Jacobs, *Tensions of a Free Press: South Africa after Apartheid* (Cambridge, Mass.: Harvard University, 1999).

3. G. Mutume, *Bringing Local Sounds to Radio* (New York: Inter Press Service, 1998).

4. B. Girard, ed. *A Passion for Radio: Radio Waves and Community* (Montreal: Black Rose Books, 1998).

5. Ibid.

6. C. Whitaker, "The Cultural Explosion," *Ebony*, August 1994.

7. K. Peart, "Township Jive," *Scholastic Update*, February 25, 1994.

8. W. Lee, "Simunye, We Are Not One: Ethnicity, Difference, and the Hip-Hoppers of Cape Town," *Race and Class* 43 (1): 29–44.

9. See "Projects—YAA 2000" at <http://www.bushradio.co.za>.

10. J. Smetherham, "HIV on Rise among Teenagers," *Cape Times*, June 14, 2002.

11. See "Projects—YAA 2000" at <http://www.bushradio.co.za>.

14

Teaching Social Studies in Botswana in the Age of HIV/AIDS

Michael Bamidele Adeyemi

In the world in 2002, Botswana, a landlocked, diamond-rich, peaceful country in southern Africa with about 1.4 million people, was the worst hit by the HIV/AIDS pandemic. Thirty-six percent of all adults (about 280,000) in what should be their most productive years (fifteen to forty-nine) were infected.[1] As a social studies teacher for many years in a Botswana junior secondary school (JSS), I have seen the impact of HIV/AIDS on the school system. The government of Botswana, in an attempt to reduce the rate of HIV infection has, through its Ministry of Education, infused AIDS-related topics into the social studies curriculum of the JSS. However, although JSS students in Botswana are highly aware of HIV/AIDS, the infection rate continues to rise.

In addition to cultural and socioeconomic factors, several behavior patterns have contributed to the pandemic, among them having unprotected sex and multiple sexual partners as well as a high prevalence of sexually transmitted diseases.[2] Among the strategies for preventing the spread of the virus are abstaining from sex, being faithful to one's partner, and using condoms.

The JSS Curriculum on HIV/AIDS

In a survey of JSS teachers in Botswana—specifically their attitude toward the ABCs of AIDS-prevention (Abstain, Be faithful, Condomize), the vast majority favored the teaching of AIDS-related topics to students, including the use of condoms, while all opposed keeping AIDS-infected students out of the schools. It was concluded that the education specialists should design an HIV/AIDS curriculum.[3]

A study of adolescents in secondary schools in Gaborone concluded that teens receive little information on HIV/AIDS; do not discuss AIDS frequently with their parents, friends, and

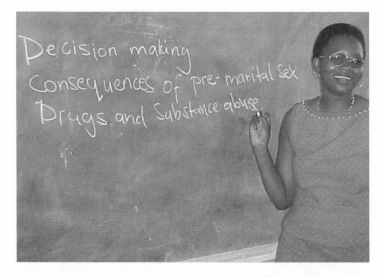

Fig. 14.1. A social studies teacher explains the importance of decision making in the prevention of HIV/AIDS to junior secondary students in Botswana. Photograph by Michael Bamidele Adeyemi. Used with permission.

significant others; and prefer to receive HIV/AIDS education from television, radio, pamphlets, and health clinics.[4] The study highlighted irrational beliefs about individuals with AIDS and the virus that causes AIDS. The authors recommended that the students should receive more information on HIV/AIDS. A need existed to encourage parents to talk more to their adolescent children, for the mass media to address the subject more, and for individuals to develop more positive attitudes toward those living with HIV and AIDS.

Sexual relationships are common in Botswana's schools; 5 percent of girls in senior secondary schools became pregnant in 1999. Noting the students' careless attitude and risky sexual behavior, the government recommended prevention strategies that included the introduction of motivational messages aimed at behavioral change, the establishment of youth-friendly centers in schools, training and support of peer educators, and prompt treatment of sexually transmitted diseases.

A 2001 report compiled by the Ministry of Education found that

- there is broad agreement among school management teams, teachers, and students, as well as among well-informed outsiders, that the current approach of "infusion and integration" of HIV/AIDS topics into the curriculum is not producing the desired changes in sexual behavior. There are also serious problems with school-based guidance and counseling services, particularly in primary schools.
- teachers are a relatively unimportant source of information on sexual and reproductive health issues for primary school students. Teachers do, though, play a significant information dissemination role in secondary schools, for both boys and girls. While major gaps in knowledge about HIV/AIDS among adolescent children exist at the primary

school level, secondary school students are relatively knowledgeable about the causes and consequences of the disease. However, this does not appear to translate into lower-risk sexual behavior.[5]

One of the nationwide surveys conducted by the Ministry of Education revealed a negative attitude among teachers with respect to the handling of HIV/AIDS issues. The following comment is typical: "Even though we teach about HIV/AIDS and the dangers of sexual intercourse, are the students really taking in the seriousness of the matter? Morality is low and promiscuity is high."[6]

The Botswana government has been trying to stem the tide of AIDS by encouraging the infusion of related topics into the syllabus. An excerpt from the Three-Year Junior Secondary Syllabus on Social Studies illustrates how seriously the government takes the pandemic: "Without injury to the subject [social studies] . . . there is an urgent need not only to make students aware of the pandemic, but also to 'work' on the behavior of students if the 'war' against the dreaded disease is to be won."[7]

Knowledge and Attitudes about HIV/AIDS among Social Studies Students

In June and July 2001, in my capacity as supervisor of teaching practice, I conducted a study among JSS students in six Botswana schools. The country was stratified into three regions: northern, central, and southern. One rural and one urban school were randomly chosen from each region.

Research instruments were administered and interviews were conducted among three hundred subjects—fifty Form 3 (ninth grade) students were randomly selected from of each of the six schools. Form 3 students were targeted because their teachers had been directed by the national social studies syllabus to present themes concerning HIV/AIDS early in the school year. For confidentiality, the schools under study were designated schools A, B (northern region, A = urban, B = rural); C, D (central region, C = urban, D = rural); and E, F (southern region, E = urban, F = rural). The average age in the total sample of 184 girls and 116 boys was fifteen and a half years. All subjects in the sample were preparing for the November 2001 Junior Certificate Examinations, which included social studies as a compulsory subject.

Many instruments (like those used by the World Health Organization and other organizations) have been used to collect data on the knowledge, attitudes, and belief about AIDS issues. Although they were available for this study, it was

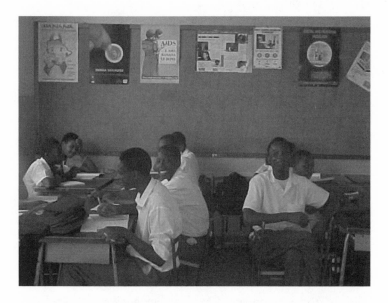

Fig. 14.2. Social studies students work in groups to discuss ways to prevent HIV/AIDS at a junior secondary school in Botswana. The AIDS posters on the wall are used as teaching aids. Photograph by Michael Bamidele Adeyemi. Used with permission.

necessary to structure an instrument more suitable for the subjects and the specific purpose of study. The present investigator therefore put simple, short questions on a piece of paper with appropriate spaces for the students to respond, after providing some demographic data.

Sample Instrument

Name of School_____

Age_____

Gender_____

Question 1: What are the causes of AIDS? (40 points)

Question 2: What differences exist between HIV and AIDS? (20 points)

Question 3: Write freely on other facts you know about HIV/AIDS. (40 points)

Question 4: What are the sources of your information on HIV/AIDS?

The answers were evaluated in a "standardized" way by judging the responses against a predetermined "ideal" response. The following performance scale was used:

70–100 points—excellent

60–69 points—very good

50–59 points—good

40–49 points—fair

Fewer than 40 points—poor

The questionnaire was distributed to the subject head in social studies to administer to the fifty students selected in each of the schools. Students were given one hour to complete the "mini-examination" and students in all six schools responded on the same day, ensuring that no one had any prior knowledge of the instrument. Based on an analysis of students' knowledge, I made recommendations on how social studies could be used as a tool to minimize the incidence of HIV/AIDS in Botswana's schools.

An examination of the six schools shows that students in urban areas have a somewhat higher level of awareness of HIV/AIDS than do their rural counterparts. The mean score for the rural schools was 50 points; for the urban schools, it was 60 points (Table 14.1). Overall, the scores show that the three hundred subjects had a fairly good awareness of HIV/AIDS.

The students' responses to the final question on the form showed the multiple sources of their knowledge about HIV/AIDS, including their ranking of the importance of each source. JSS students, whether from rural or urban settings, obtain most of their information about HIV/AIDS from social studies classes, but radio and talking with friends, peers, and parents and relatives are also significant sources of information (Table 14.2).

Although the countrywide survey conducted by the Ministry of Education on HIV/AIDS depicts a high level of awareness among students, there is broad agreement among school management teams, teachers, and students, as well as among well-informed outsiders, that the current "infusion and integration"

Table 14-1
Awareness of HIV/AIDS among
Rural and Urban Junior Secondary Students

Level of Performance	Rural Schools (n = 150)	Urban Schools (n = 150)
Excellent (70–100 points)	5%	17%
Very Good (60–69 points)	19%	35%
Good (50–59 points)	30%	33%
Fair (40–49 points)	20%	8%
Poor (fewer than 40 points)	26%	7%
Mean Score	50 points	60 points

Table 14.2

Sources of Awareness of HIV/AIDS among
Rural and Urban Junior Secondary Students

Source of Awareness	Rural Schools (n = 150)		Urban Schools (n = 150)	
	Percent	Source Rank	Percent	Source Rank
Social studies class	57%	1	85%	1
Peers and friends	39%	2	68%	4
Radio	30%	3	83%	2
Pamphlets and newspapers	21%	4	47%	5
Clinics and hospitals	18%	5	33%	8
Churches and mosques	15%	6	30%	9
Parents and relatives	13%	7	35%	7
Television	7%	8 (tie)	81%	3
NGOs	7%	8 (tie)	20%	10
Guest speakers in school	6%	10	39%	6
Other sources	3%	11	17%	11

NOTE: percentages total more than one hundred because students listed multiple
sources.

of HIV/AIDS topics into the curriculum is not producing the
desired changes in sexual behavior.

A study by the World Health Organization, jointly conducted with the University of Botswana and the Ministry of
Education, also found a high level of awareness of the pandemic but "careless" attitudinal behavior with respect to prevention.[8] An earlier study concluded that junior secondary
students have more negative attitudes toward prevention
strategies than their senior secondary counterparts.[9]

The current situation leaves social studies teachers in a
dilemma. On the one hand there are many intelligent students
who know the intricacies in terms of the causes, effects, incur-
ability, and prevention strategies for HIV/AIDS. On the other
hand the same students refuse to abide by the rules of preven-

tion. Typical of the responses I encountered during my interviews is their preference for unsafe sex over the use of a condom: "Using a condom is like eating candy with the wrapper left on. It won't taste sweet unless it's unwrapped."

Revamping the Social Studies Curriculum

Social studies, as a core subject at the JSS level, has a role to play in reducing the incidence of HIV/AIDS in junior secondary schools in Botswana by addressing these negative attitudes. The social studies teacher can strike a balance among the rational, emotional, and physical domains of teaching. The findings of the present study suggest that social studies teachers should place greater emphasis on the affective (emotional) domain when teaching topics dealing with HIV/AIDS. This should be a consideration when designing the social studies syllabus.

Teachers should use techniques that will examine students' attitudes. The social studies syllabus should emphasize the use of moral dilemmas in teaching about HIV/AIDS issues in the classroom. Teachers could use stories and dramas of men infecting their wives or boyfriends infecting their girlfriends with the virus. For example, my students listened attentively to the following story about a boy who repeatedly refused to use condoms:

> There is a very handsome boy in a village not far from here. He is also very brilliant and has several girlfriends. He has sex with them without taking any precaution. He insists on unsafe sex every time. Eventually he becomes infected with the HIV virus. He now has a new HIV-negative girlfriend who insists on safe sex. The boy refuses.

I asked my students, "If you were in the same situation with the new girlfriend, what would you do?" Answers to this question may vary, as it poses a moral dilemma. The social studies teacher should use this type of moral dilemma (or role play) to equip his or her students with the skills to make informed and reasoned choices. Such dramatic situations in sex/AIDS education can reinforce the positive cultural values of the society. This might change their lifestyles.

I further suggest that elders in the society teach children about moral aspects of HIV/AIDS. Parents and relatives need to talk to their children, while community and religious leaders should be invited to speak in schools. To arouse the feelings of the students, guest speakers can relate time-honored stories that reinforce our values system. Emphasis on self-discipline is necessary if the rate of infection is to be slowed. Topics related to self-discipline and the ability to make reasoned decisions should be part of the day-to-day activities in schools.

Discussions on how to change from irresponsible to responsible behavior should form a significant part of educational television and radio broadcasts to schools. Video and audio programs recorded by the media should be made available to social studies teachers for use in classrooms. Finally, the social studies curriculum should be revised from time to time to include emerging issues related to the continuing war against HIV/AIDS.

Notes

1. UNAIDS, *Global HIV/AIDS and STD Surveillance: Epidemiological Fact Sheets by Country*, <http://www.unaids.org>, 2000.

2. Ministry of Health, *Seventh Sentinel Surveillance in Botswana* (Gaborone: AIDS/STD Unit, 1998).

3. M. B. Adeyemi and R. Tabulawa, "AIDS and Related Issues: The Views of Junior Secondary Teachers in Botswana," *Educational Studies* 19, 2 (1993): 227–34.

4. A. A. Alao, L. W. Odirile, and I. Kandji-Murangi, "Knowledge, Attitudes, and Beliefs Related to HIV/AIDS among Adolescents in Secondary Schools in Gaborone, Botswana," research project funded by National Institute of Development Research and Documentation, Centre for Graduate Studies and Research in the Faculty of Education, University of Botswana on behalf of the Swedish Agency for Research Cooperation in Developing Countries (SAREC), 1995.

5. B. Chilisa and P. Bennell with Botswana, Ministry of Education, and United Kingdom, Department for International Development, *The Impact of HIV/AIDS on Primary and Secondary Education in Botswana: Developing a Comprehensive Strategic Response* (London: Department for International Development, 2001).

6. Ibid.

7. Republic of Botswana, *Three-Year Junior Secondary Syllabus (Social Studies)* (Gaborone: Curriculum Development Division, Department of Curriculum Development and Evaluation, Ministry of Education, 1996).

8. University of Botswana, Ministry of Health, and World Health Organization, *A Study of Knowledge, Attitude, and Behavioral Aspects of HIV/AIDS among Students of the University of Botswana* (Gaborone: University of Botswana, 1999).

9. Alao, Odirile, and Kandji-Murangi, "Knowledge, Attitudes, and Beliefs."

15

Communication Strategies for Confronting AIDS

Empowering the Children of Africa

Arvind Singhal

The introduction to the present volume cited singer Oliver Mtukudzi's question to the youth of Zimbabwe about the AIDS crisis: "What shall we do?" In the context of Zimbabwe, where 45 percent of the children under the age of five are HIV positive and where one of every two fifteen-year-olds is likely to die of AIDS, Mtukudzi's question embodies both a national crisis and a continent's anguish.

So what shall we do? While there are no short-cuts or simple formulas for tackling AIDS, the discourse of what can be done is framed in the context of courage, hope, and possibilities. While the world is now more than ten years into the HIV/AIDS crisis with no promising vaccine in sight, and with relatively few effective and sustainable prevention programs, several key lessons have been learned about confronting the pandemic.

I discuss these lessons from my vantage point as a communications scholar interested in overcoming the communicative challenges presented by HIV/AIDS: silence, denial, blame, stigma, prejudice, and discrimination. McGeary aptly summarized these challenges: "The victims don't cry out. Doctors and obituaries do not give the killer its name. Families recoil in shame. Leaders shirk responsibility. The stubborn silence heralds victory for the disease: denial cannot keep the virus at bay."[1]

How can communication strategies address these challenges—strategically, creatively, and compassionately? I organize the response to this question around four key communicative lessons. Perhaps some of these lessons can empower the children of Africa as they face the relentless onslaught of AIDS.

Lesson 1: "When the Lion Comes, Make a Loud Shout"

In April 2002, during the International Conference on HIV/AIDS and the African Child, held at Ohio University, I picked up a copy of *African Recovery*, which featured a story on how Uganda is facing the AIDS "lion." In this story, Ugandan president Yoweri Museveni goaded his fellow African heads of state to personally lead the charge on AIDS. He said: "When a lion comes to the village, you don't make a small alarm. You make a very loud one. When I knew of AIDS, I said we must shout and shout and shout and shout."[2]

Museveni's use of the word *shout* signifies a key communication strategy to confront AIDS. Shouting signifies a mustering of political leadership, a call to action, and, perhaps more important, the need to be heard loud and clear amid a cacophony of confusion or, as some have suggested, a deafening veil of silence. Museveni believes that his fellow "village chiefs" need to confront the AIDS lion head-on as the beast continues to decimate the village stock, especially the most vulnerable young ones. Doing anything less is unpardonable.

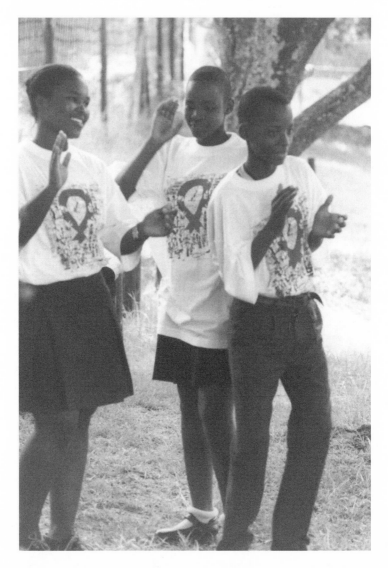

Fig. 15.1. High school students in KwaZulu-Natal Province, South Africa, during an interactive theater performance designed to break the community's silence on AIDS. Johns Hopkins University Center for Communication Programs. Photograph by Patrick L. Coleman, JHU/CCP. Used with permission.

In our communication courses, we discuss the importance of analyzing communication phenomena by posing the question, Who says what to whom in what context and with what effect? Once again, Museveni's follow-up remarks to his fellow African chiefs reflect a strategic grasp of communicative action: "When a district health officer comes to address a village meeting, 20 people show up. When Museveni addresses a rally, 20,000 show up. That's the time to pass the AIDS message." "The top leadership needs to supervise the AIDS war."[3]

Breaking the silence on AIDS by "shouting" loudly allows a nation, a community, or a family to step up from words to deeds. Uganda, for instance, has mobilized its civil society—schools, churches, mosques, mass media—to spread the word on AIDS. Wherever people congregate, the "village chief"—whether a political, educational, religious, or community leader—has a key role to play in confronting AIDS through leadership, action, and compassion. In Uganda's public schools, headmasters talk about AIDS in student assemblies. In its mosques, imams talk about AIDS during congregational prayers, home visits, and community ceremonies.

The timing of the shout is critical too. During a visit to Nairobi in 2001, I noticed that Kenyan president Daniel arap Moi called attention to the pandemic in every speech he gave, whatever the topic and whoever the audience. The president, when inaugurating a new kindergarten, urged his audience of small children to avoid becoming infected with HIV. Earlier, in the 1980s, Moi went through several years of denial, insisting that there was no AIDS in Kenya. Today, the Ministry of Health estimates that seven hundred Kenyans die every day from AIDS. The lesson from Kenya is that the shouting needs to begin in earnest, and early; the delay can be measured only in lost lives.

Lesson 2: Frame the Shout:
Setting the Media, Public, and Policy Agenda

But how does an issue like AIDS get on the national agenda? How does the shout rise above the deafening silence of apathy and inaction? What role can the mass media, especially journalists, play in amplifying the shout? How can the stifled needs and aspirations of children infected and affected by HIV/ AIDS be voiced to influence the mass media, public, and policy discourse?

African countries need a cadre of child-friendly journalists and perhaps an agency that monitors media coverage of children. Here, ANDI's (Agência de Notícias dos Direitos da Infância) experience in Brazil is noteworthy. ANDI is a news organization that proactively monitors media coverage of children, with a special emphasis on HIV/AIDS. ANDI regularly content analyzes some forty Brazilian magazines and newspapers to gauge how HIV/AIDS is covered. A report is then published that details what the media *are* doing with respect to HIV/AIDS, what they are *not* doing, and what they *should* be doing.[4] ANDI then conducts training sessions for journalists on AIDS reporting and provides them with a manual that includes contact information for HIV/AIDS officials at the federal, state, and municipal levels plus a list of NGOs working in this field. Reporters are trained in how to compassionately report on people living with HIV and AIDS, stimulate public debate, and reduce the stigma and homophobia that often accompanies the disease.

ANDI's biggest accomplishment, in my opinion, is the creation of a cadre of 250 child-friendly journalists in Brazil who regularly report accurately and compassionately on children's issues. ANDI believes that when a reporter frames a story from the perspective of children, the story takes on a human face, is engaging to the reader, and allows for issues to be examined in the context of future possibilities. For instance, an outbreak of cholera in a Brazilian favela might emphasize the role of the health sector in immunizing children against preventable diseases.

Cynthia Garda, a child-friendly journalist (an honor bestowed on her by ANDI), recalled her first story on AIDS orphans in Brazil: "When I got in touch with ANDI, they told me which NGOs and government offices to possibly contact in the local area. . . . They also made available to me, through their clipping service, all previous articles published in Brazil on AIDS orphans." Garda also told me how ANDI helped change the face of AIDS in the Brazilian media: "Previously HIV-positive children were not shown in Brazilian newspapers. Their faces were hidden or covered. And yesterday there were six smiling children on the front page of the national newspaper, and the headline said, 'We Are Positive.'"[5]

ANDI monitors media coverage of children and HIV/AIDS on a regular basis so that it can track the quantitative and qualitative changes in AIDS reporting in Brazil. By showing these results to journalists and training them in accurate HIV/AIDS reporting, ANDI initiates and influences the public and policy debates about AIDS in Brazil.

ANDI also knows that when AIDS is humanized, news reports catch the public's attention, people believe that AIDS is an important social problem, and it climbs to prominence on the national agenda.[6] ANDI has learned that factual indicators like rates of HIV infection often do not play an important role in setting the media agenda.[7] In the United States the issue of HIV/AIDS lay dormant for four years (AIDS was first diagnosed in 1981), during which time more than twenty thousand people died of the disease. The U.S. mass media were mostly silent. However, when film star Rock Hudson disclosed his HIV status in 1985, the issue of AIDS was humanized and rapidly climbed the U.S. media agenda (subsequently stirring the public and policy agendas). And in South Africa, despite several years of galloping HIV infections, the media's shout on AIDS was barely audible until AIDS got its public face—the courageous child Nkosi Johnson (see chapter 6).

"Poster people" not only set media, public, and policy agendas, they show that people living with HIV/AIDS are individuals just like everyone else.

Lesson 3: Create Safe, Nonstigmatized Communicative Spaces

As noted previously, from a communications perspective HIV/AIDS is not merely a biological illness but a disease of ignorance and intolerance. If the mass media profile it as a disease only of gays, intravenous drug users, and commercial sex workers, it perpetuates stigma—which is every bit as dangerous as the virus itself. Stigma implies dying every second, a type of living death.[8] AIDS stigma evokes negative reactions—denial, shame, fear, anger, prejudice, and discrimination—that manifest themselves in interpersonal and group relationships. Hence, communication strategies need to be at the heart of all efforts to overcome the stigma of HIV and AIDS.

Let's consider the case of Pink Triangle Malaysia (PTM), a nongovernmental organization that operates an innovative outreach program targeted at intravenous drug users (IDUs) in Chow Kit, a poor red-light community in Kuala Lumpur, the nation's capital. PTM creatively uses space to reduce stigma and prejudice.[9] A culturally sensitive research protocol to assess the clients' needs, prior to launching the PTM program, pointed to the importance of creating an Ikhlas ("sincere" or "compassionate") Community Center (ICC), a safe space where the IDUs would feel comfortable about dropping in. The ICC provides meals to IDUs, medical care and treatment, referrals to hospitals and drug treatment centers, counseling and psychological support, access to condoms and other risk-reduction services, and job referrals. Clean facilities are also provided so that drug users can bathe, wash their clothes, and maintain personal hygiene.

The IDUs participate in running these ICC activities: They cook and clean, serve as outreach workers and volunteer counselors, and carry out administrative work. This involvement helps them take ownership of the Ikhlas project and builds their self-esteem. The IDUs of the ICC routinely liaise with volunteer groups from hospitals, nursing schools, the corporate sector, and colleges and thus feel more accepted by the general community. Their active involvement also makes Pink Triangle Malaysia's Ikhlas program highly successful and cost-effective.

The Ikhlas program holds at least two key lessons for African children and communities as they confront AIDS. First, it highlights the important role of locally based NGOs in creating culturally responsive community-based interventions. Second, it reinforces the importance of creating nonstigmatized, nonjudgmental spaces where adults and children, including those affected by HIV/AIDS, can feel nurtured, loved, and safe.

Y-Centres (short for Youth Centre) in South Africa are nonclinical, friendly spaces where youth can mingle, learn, and play in a safe community environment.[10] loveLife, an organization that works with youth to reduce teenage pregnancy, prevent HIV infections, and build a sense of community, has established over a dozen Y-Centres across South Africa. Each Y-Centre provides youth a multipurpose recreational center equipped with basketball courts, a sexual health education center, and a counseling facility.

Y-Centres offer basketball clinics , and NBA-style championships foster a competitive spirit.[11] The basketball clinics go beyond teaching how to pass and shoot; they teach young boys and girls about lifeskills, about taking care of their bodies, and about sexual responsibility. loveLife also holds loveGames, a nationwide mini-olympiad in which youth compete in popular local games such as soccer, rugby, and track and field. Through its sports and educational programs, Y-Centres train youth members to serve as HIV/AIDS peer educators in their communities. Each Y-Centre comes equipped with a mobile broadcasting unit, which empowers youth by allowing them to hear their voices on the air when covering local sports events.

Safe spaces for children can also be created in other normally threatening environments. For instance, courts in Zimbabwe modified their judicial proceedings to protect the rights of sexually assaulted children.[12] Before the establishment of the child-friendly courts, children faced hostile questioning in regular courtrooms, face-to-face with their adult abusers. Intimidated by the courtroom atmosphere, they often broke down, refused to speak, or had great difficulty in describing the sexual act. Without their testimony, the accused was often acquitted.

In the child-friendly court system, when a sexual offence complaint is initiated on behalf of a child, the Zimbabwean police and social welfare officers work with the child to reduce their physical and emotional trauma.[13] Children now give courtroom testimony sitting in a separate room through closed-circuit television. A trained intermediary relays the court's question to the child in gentle language that the child can understand. The child can also use male and female dolls to demonstrate the sexual act without describing it. By 2000 every province in Zimbabwe had at least one child-friendly court.

Comfortable spaces can also be created virtually—for instance, through the Internet and telephone help-lines. In 2001 the Romanian Society for Education on Contraception and Sexuality launched a website to provide information and counseling to youth about STDs, unwanted pregnancies, and HIV/

AIDS.[14] It soon became one of Romania's most popular youth websites, attracting over a hundred thousand hits during its first year.[15] A medical doctor and a support staff provide confidential advice to visitors. The website also offers youth chat groups, a peer education forum, and links to other locally available HIV/AIDS services in Romania. The anonymity of the virtual interaction promotes an open discussion of HIV/AIDS topics.

Such websites—accessible from schools, libraries, and telecenters, designed locally with culturally sensitive content, and staffed by compassionate counselors— can provide comfortable, nonstigmatized, virtual spaces for African adolescents to express themselves. HIV/AIDS telephone help-lines, much like their Internet counterparts, can also provide a confidential, nonjudgmental, nonembarrassing virtual space that is highly responsive to the individualized needs of callers.[16]

Lesson 4: Redefine the Problem: Harnessing Cultural Undercurrents

How an issue is socially constructed determines, to a large extent, how it will be approached. In the African context, communication strategies have mainly constructed HIV/AIDS as a life-threatening disease to be feared—a disease that results from promiscuous and deviant behaviors of others.[17] Hence, past communication approaches have mostly been antisex, antipleasure, and fear inducing. While sexuality involves pleasure, communication strategies have rarely viewed sex as play, as adventure, as fun, as fantasy, as giving, as sharing, as spirituality, or as ritual.[18]

It is not surprising that most HIV/AIDS intervention programs are flying blind and culturally rudderless.[19] Anthropologist Richard Parker argues that the "erotic experience" is often situated in acts of "sexual transgression," that is, the deliberate undermining, in private, of public norms.[20] The common Brazilian expression *Entre quarto paredes, tudo pode acontecer* ("Within four walls, anything can happen") signifies how the erotic experience—for both men and women—lies in the freedom of such hidden moments.[21] This social and cultural construction of eroticism may explain why a well-to-do man with a happy, stable marriage and children may play sugar daddy to an adolescent girl or visit a commercial sex worker. Within four walls, such a partner may perform a range of sexual acts that a "proper" wife would shun.

At a 2000 UNAIDS meeting in Geneva, a representative from Kenya talked about how young schoolgirls in his country rendered sexual favors to urban middle-class and affluent men in the middle and upper classes (sugar daddies) in exchange for the 3Cs: cash, cell phones, and cars. Sugar daddies initiate the seduction process by asking young girls: "Let me buy you chicken and chips" or "Let me give you a lift in my car." Rates of HIV infection among young girls in Kenya are six times higher than for young boys, and exploitation by sugar daddies is largely responsible for this difference. Ethnographic research with schoolgirls in Kenya has shown that they were well aware of the high risks they faced in contracting HIV but were willing to take their chances.[22] Why say no to such glamorous adventures when the alternative is to struggle through school and college, find a job, and, once married, attend to domestic chores and reproductive roles?

In this case, it is important for communicators to understand the strong cultural undercurrents about masculine sexuality in Kenya. It is important to understand that sugar daddies bed young girls as trophies and that cash, cell phones, and cars are symbols of power, prestige, and modernity for all Kenyans, especially adolescent girls. In such situations, cleverly crafted, individual-directed messages such as "Stay away from sugar daddies" or "Stay away from schoolgirls" are likely to be ineffective.

In the past most communication interventions have focused on changing the behaviors of individuals—such as that of sugar daddies or of adolescent girls at high risk for HIV infection. Metaphorically speaking, they have been trying to analyze and influence the bobbing of individual corks as they float in a stream of water. In the future, they should focus on understanding and redirecting the strong undercurrents that determine where the cork clusters end up along the shoreline.[23] In order to do so, communication programmers must be immersed in local waters and understand the undercurrents. They should value indigenous knowledge in designing, developing, and implementing culturally sensitive, participatory communication interventions.

Culture as an Ally

Communication strategists have also been guilty of viewing culture as static and mistakenly looking upon people's health beliefs as cultural barriers. This conceptual coupling of culture and barriers needs to be exposed, deconstructed, and reconstructed so that new positive cultural linkages can be forged.[24] Attributes of a culture that are helpful for confronting AIDS should be identified and harnessed.[25]

For instance, the cultural attributes of the Nguni people in southern Africa reveal points of entry for communicating HIV/AIDS behavior change. Among the Nguni, at the onset of puberty a youth's sexual education is usually delegated to an aunt or uncle. Cultural emphasis is placed on sexual abstinence.[26] A strong taboo exists against bringing one's family name to disrepute. *Ukusoma* (a Zulu term for nonpenetrative sex) is commonly practiced, both to preserve virginity and to prevent pregnancy. The woman keeps her thighs close to-gether while the man finds sexual release. Other groups use a bent elbow for a similar purpose. Similar nonpenetrative sex practices exist among certain groups in Ethiopia (commonly referred to as brushing), the Kikuyu in Kenya, and other groups.

In Kenya, MYWO (Maendeleo ya Wanawake Organization), a women's development organization, and PATH (Program for Alternative Technology in Health) created an alternative ceremony for young girls facing female circumcision. Called Ntanira na Mugambo (loosely, circumcision through words), this approach was mooted when a group of Kenyan mothers sought alternative ways to usher their daughters into woman-hood.[27] This community-based approach, which preserves all rituals of the original ceremony except the circumcision, in-cludes song, education, celebration, feasting, and a week of seclusion for the young girls (to coincide with the traditional healing period). During this week, each young woman works with a female mentor who teaches her about sexuality, rela-tionships, sexually transmitted diseases (including AIDS), and reproductive anatomy. To date, some five thousand girls have participated in these ceremonies, thus avoiding the risk of HIV infection during circumcision ceremonies.

Similarly, virginity testing is regaining popularity in South Africa.[28] Goaded by NGOs, various community-based move-ments have sprung up that work with mothers of adolescent girls to reinstate such traditional Zulu rites. Mothers believe that if their daughters remain virgins before marriage, their risk of contracting HIV will be substantially reduced (if not delayed).

Local, vernacular-based communication art forms are also important tools in addressing HIV/AIDS. Most HIV/AIDS communication campaigns in Africa have undervalued tradi-tional oral communication channels and the strength of aural comprehension. In African countries the oral tradition—

proverbs, adages, riddles, folklore, and storytelling—is rich in visual imagery and is the basis on which learning is founded.[29] The narrative tradition offers the potential of cultural expression, particularly words of advice and encouragement, that are often couched in adage, allegory, and metaphor.[30]

Furthermore, communication interventions fare better if scientific explanations of health issues are couched in local contexts of understanding. Such context-based explanations are called syncretic explanations.[31] A diarrhea prevention campaign in northern Nigeria illustrates the importance of providing syncretic explanations. When missionaries in Nigeria were alarmed about the number of infant deaths due to diarrhea, they tried to teach mothers about water boiling. The mothers were told that their children died because of little animals in the water and that boiling the water could kill these animals. Talk of invisible animals in water was met with skepticism. Babies kept on dying. Finally, a visiting anthropologist suggested a solution. There were, he said, "evil spirits in the water; boil the water and you could see them going away, bubbling out to escape the heat."[32] This message had the desired effect, and infant mortality due to diarrhea dropped sharply.

In essence, communication strategies to confront AIDS in Africa must view culture as an ally. Indigenous contexts of understanding, folk traditions, and magico-religious myths—all are potential tools in the fight against AIDS.

Important lessons have been learned about the role of communication strategies in breaking the silence on AIDS and framing media, public, and policy debates in ways that stimulate ground-based, community-centered action. Communication can be used both as a scalpel and a sledgehammer in the fight against AIDS. As a Buddhist monk noted, "HIV/AIDS is like a huge rock in society. Only if everyone in society keeps breaking the rock into smaller pieces will it eventually become dust."[33]

Notes

This chapter draws upon Arvind Singhal and Everett M. Rogers, *Combating AIDS: Communication Strategies in Action* (Thousand Oaks, Calif.: Sage Publications, 2003).

1. Johanna McGeary, "Death Stalks a Continent," *Time*, February 12, 2001, 36–45.

2. In Gumisai Mutume, "African Leaders Declare War on AIDS," *Africa Recovery* 14, 1 (2001): 21.

3. Ibid.

4. Singhal and Rogers, *Combating AIDS*.

5. Cynthia Garda, interview by author, Brasilia, Brazil, March 15, 2001.

6. James W. Dearing and Everett M. Rogers, *Agenda-Setting* (Thousand Oaks, Calif.: Sage Publications, 1996).

7. Singhal and Rogers, *Combating AIDS*.

8. Ibid.

9. UNAIDS, *Comfort and Hope: Six Case Studies on Mobilizing Family and Community Care for and by People with HIV/AIDS* (Geneva: UNAIDS, 1999).

10. Singhal and Rogers, *Combating AIDS*.

11. Lungi Morrison, interview by author, Johannesburg, South Africa, June 13, 2001.

12. UNAIDS, *AIDS Epidemic Update, December 2000*, <http://www.unaids.org/wac/2000/wad00/files/WAD_epidemic_report.htm>, 2000.

13. Ibid.

14. <http://www.sexdex.ro>

15. Dan Dionisie, "HIV/AIDS Counseling for Teens in Romania," *Choices* 10, 4 (2001): 19.

16. Mukesh Kapila and Maryan J. Pye, "The European Response to AIDS," in *AIDS Prevention through Education: A World View*, ed. Jaime Sepulveda, Harvey Fineberg, and Jonathan Mann (New York: Oxford University Press, 1992), 199–236.

17. Vera Paiva, "Sexuality, AIDS, and Gender Norms among Brazilian Teenagers," in *Culture and Sexual Risk: Anthropological Perspectives on AIDS*, ed. Han ten Brummelheis and Gilbert Herdt (Amsterdam: Gordon and Breach, 1995), 79–96.

18. Ralph Bolton, "Rethinking Anthropology: The Study of AIDS," in *Culture and Sexual Risk: Anthropological Perspectives on AIDS*, ed. Han ten Brummelheis and Gilbert Herdt (Amsterdam: Gordon and Breach, 1995), 285–314.

19. Singhal and Rogers, *Combating AIDS*.

20. Richard Parker, *Bodies, Pleasures, and Passions: Sexual Culture in Contemporary Brazil* (Boston: Beacon Press, 1991); Herbert Daniel and Richard Parker, *Sexuality, Politics, and AIDS in Brazil* (London: Falmer Press, 1993).

21. Daniel and Parker, *Sexuality, Politics, and AIDS*.

22. Singhal and Rogers, *Combating AIDS*.

23. A. J. McMichael, "The Health of Persons, Populations, and Planets: Epidemiology Comes Full Circle," *Epidemiology* 6 (1995): 636–63.

24. Collins O. Airhihenbuwa and Rafael Obregon, "A Critical Assessment of Theories/Models Used in Health Communication for HIV/AIDS," *Journal of Health Communication* 5 (2000): 5–15.

25. Collins O. Airhihenbuwa, *Health and Culture: Beyond the Western Paradigm* (Thousand Oaks, Calif.: Sage Publications, 1995).

26. Arvind Singhal, *HIV/AIDS in Communication for Behavior and Social Change: Program Experiences, Examples, and the Way Forward* (Geneva: UNAIDS, 2001).

27. See <http://www.path.org/resources/press-room.htm>.

28. McGeary, "Death Stalks a Continent."

29. Collins O. Airhihenbuwa, "Of Culture and Multiverse: Renouncing 'The Universal Truth' in Health," *Journal of Health Education* 30, 5 (1999): 267–73.

30. Arvind Singhal and Everett M. Rogers, *Entertainment-Education: A Communication Strategy for Social Change* (Mahwah, N.J.: Lawrence Erlbaum Associates, 1999).

31. T. Barnett and P. Blaikie, *AIDS in Africa: Its Present and Future Impact* (New York: Guilford Press, 1992).

32. B. Okri, *The Famished Road* (New York: Oxford University Press, 1991), 134–35.

33. Sommai Punnyakamo, "Coming to Terms with Truth," *Choices* 10, 4 (2001): 24.

Contributors

Michael Bamidele Adeyemi teaches social studies education in the Department of Languages and Social Sciences Education at the University of Botswana, Gaborone. He earned an M.A. in education from the University of Ife (now Obafemi Awolowo University) in Nigeria and an M.S. and Ph.D. in social studies education from Indiana University. His research focuses on the theory and practice of social studies and global education. His articles have appeared in many international journals and he has edited and written many volumes on social studies education.

Mira Aghi was one of the pioneers of the tradition of formative research for program development in India. She has trained researchers in South Asia, eastern and southern Africa, and South America in qualitative research methodologies for over twenty years. She earned her Ph.D. in psychology from Loyola University, Chicago, and has served as principal researcher for communication technology projects in the United States, South Asia, and Africa. She was also senior program officer with Canada's International Development Research Centre. She is presently working with WHO on a global tobacco use intervention aimed at women.

Janet Amegatcher grew up and was educated in Ghana. She trained as a teacher at the University of Cape Coast, Ghana.

After teaching for four years, she returned to the Ghana School of Law to earn a degree—motivated by a strong desire to fight for the rights of the weak and underprivileged. She is currently a human rights advocate.

Aadielah Anderson has an interest in health promotion and works with the Soul City Institute of Health and Development Communication in South Africa. She is presently responsible for developing and managing the second *Soul Buddyz* series. She has served as a consultant to the BBC World Service Trust's HIV/AIDS media project in India.

Tanja Bosch is a doctoral student in the School of Telecommunications at Ohio University. She holds an M.A. in Communication and Development Studies from Ohio University. Tanja has worked as a production assistant in the local film industry in Cape Town, as a programmer and producer for Bush Radio, and as a producer and consultant to Roots FM in Jamaica and UNESCO in Trinidad and Barbados. She is currently working on a dissertation on the role of community radio in postapartheid South Africa, at Bush Radio in Cape Town.

Rachel Carnegie earned an M.A. in education from Sussex University. In Bhutan she was health education program adviser with Save the Children. In Bangladesh she was health education consultant to a range of NGOs and creative consultant to UNICEF for the Meena Communication Initiative. Since 1994 she has been a core adviser to the Sara Communication Initiative in Africa and is currently a consultant on lifeskills education, health promotion, and participatory communication. Recent work includes a source book on female genital mutilation and a review of the lifeskills education initiative in Uganda.

Alicia Skinner Cook, professor in the Department of Human Development and Family Studies at Colorado State University, is a licensed psychologist with an interest in intervention programs for the bereaved. In Kenya she helped design a needs assessment instrument for children affected by HIV/AIDS and was a senior technical consultant on two USAID-funded projects. She has published more than forty articles, including work on the ethics of bereavement research. She has developed and taught courses on death, dying, and grief and has coauthored *Dying and Grieving* (2d ed.) and a book for therapists and counselors, *Helping the Bereaved,* that is used in many countries.

Farid Esack is a Muslim theologian who played a leading role in the struggle against apartheid. He currently serves as trustee of the Treatment Action Campaign and is director of Positive Muslims, an organization working with Muslims who are HIV positive.

Susan Fox has an M.A. in international relations and is currently project manager at the Centre for AIDS Development Research and Evaluation in Johannesburg.

Janet Julia Fritz is a professor in the Department of Human Development and Family Studies at Colorado State University. Her research and teaching have focused on program evaluation, risk and resilience, childhood stress and coping, and cross-cultural variations within developmental processes. Her work with evaluating early intervention programs designed for teachers, parents, community members, and children and adolescents is summarized in *A Systems Approach to the Early Prevention of Problem Behaviors.* She has also worked with colleagues in Kenya on the needs of children and families in coping with the high incidence of HIV/AIDS.

Aiah A. Gbakima is a medical researcher at Johns Hopkins University School of Hygiene and Public Health and teaches at Morgan State University. He is editor-in-chief of the *Journal of Environmental Assessment and Management,* a peer review scientist for the *American Journal of Tropical Medicine and Hygiene,* and a board member of the International Society of African Scientists.

Sue Goldstein, a public health specialist with a special interest in health promotion and health communication, qualified as a medical practitioner at the University of the Witwatersrand and practiced primary health care in Soweto and Alexandra townships in South Africa. Since 1995 she has worked with the Soul City Institute of Health and Development Communication in many roles, from managing the *Soul City* series to researching, developing, and managing the children's series *Soul Buddyz.* She has written a book on health promotion in South Africa and cofounded the South African journal *Critical Health.*

W. Stephen Howard, a sociologist by training with a Ph.D. from Michigan State University, is an associate professor of transcultural studies in education at Ohio University and director of African Studies. In 1998 he founded the Institute for the African Child at Ohio University, an interdisciplinary teaching and research initiative to seek a place in academia for the world's most marginalized populations. He has published on social movements and Islamic society in Africa, rural development, and educational change. His writing, research, and teaching in Africa cover Chad, Egypt, Ghana, Niger, Nigeria, South Africa, Sudan, Swaziland, and Tanzania.

Garth Japhet received his M.D. from the University of the Witwatersrand, South Africa, and has worked in several urban and rural clinics in South Africa. His clinical experience led him to the mass media to promote health and development. In 1991 he cofounded Soul City, an NGO that uses mass media to promote health, and presently serves as its executive director.

Michael J. Kelly has been involved with education in Zambia since 1956. Since 1975, he has served as dean of education, deputy vice-chancellor, and professor of education at the University of Zambia. He has become increasingly involved in analyzing, documenting, and making presentations on the potential for education to overcome the HIV/AIDS pandemic in Africa.

Neill McKee earned an M.S. in communication from Florida State University and is senior technical advisor for HIV/AIDS at the Johns Hopkins University Center for Communication Programs. He worked previously with the Canadian volunteer agency CUSO, Canada's International Development Research Centre, and has had UNICEF postings in Bangladesh, Nairobi, and Uganda. He is the originator of the Meena and Sara Communication Initiatives and a cofounder of Visualisation in Participatory Programmes. He is author of *Social Mobilization and Social Marketing in Developing Communities* and chief editor and contributing author for *Involving People, Evolving Behaviour.*

Marda Mustapha is a doctoral candidate in political science at Northern Arizona University. His research centers on international health policy, development, democracy, and conflict studies.

Gladys Mutangadura is an economics affairs officer with the United Nations Economic Commission for Africa. She holds a Ph.D. in agricultural economics from Virginia Polytechnic and

State University. Her research interests center around agricultural development, gender, poverty, health, and the socioeconomic impacts of the HIV/AIDS epidemic in sub-Saharan Africa. She has written several articles on the responses of rural households and communities to the HIV/AIDS pandemic.

Rose Mwonya is a professor in the Division of Research and Extension at Egerton University, Kenya. She has lectured on the social aspects of contemporary health and has been a trainer for workshops on social behavior and the prevention of STDs. A former Fulbright scholar, she has been a gender consultant on numerous projects in East Africa and currently is coordinator of student counseling through the Egerton University Health Project. She was also facilitator for health and gender awareness workshops for secondary schools in Nakuru District, Kenya. Through a farmer-to-farmer program, she helped assess the impact of HIV/AIDS on agricultural communities in western Kenya.

Prisca N. Nemapare is chief program officer for the Zienzele Foundation in Zimbabwe and served as visiting professor at Ritsumeikan University in Kyoto, Japan, while this chapter was written. She taught at Ohio University (1982–98), where her research and teaching interests centered around nutrition and maternal and child health issues. She is author of three books and several journal articles.

Warren Parker is director of the Centre for AIDS Development Research and Evaluation in Johannesburg and an HIV/AIDS communication specialist. He has worked and consulted for NGOs and governmental groups in the field of development and HIV/AIDS in South Africa and internationally, and he has directed and overseen a wide range of communication campaigns and activities. His research includes participatory development communication with youth and HIV/AIDS communication for youth and children in South Africa.

Amy S. Patterson earned a Ph.D. in political science from Indiana University and teaches political science at Calvin College, Grand Rapids, Michigan. She has published in several journals and edited volumes, including *The Journal of Modern African Studies, Africa Today, African Studies Review,* and *PS: Political Science and Politics.* Her research interests include African democratization, gender and development, and the politics of HIV/AIDS in Africa.

Yegan Pillay is assistant director in the Office for Institutional Equity at Ohio University. He is licensed by the South African Medical and Dental Council as a psychologist and is licensed as a professional clinical counselor by the Counselor and Social Worker Board of Ohio.

Esca Scheepers earned an M.A. in critical psychology from Rhodes University, South Africa. She is a research methodologist specializing in the evaluation of mass media health and development communication. She has consulted on, managed, and conducted various forms of evaluation research in both mainstream and community media environments. She is currently involved in the evaluation of the Soul City Regional Programme in Africa.

Nuzhat Shahzadi holds an M.P.H. with specialization in health education. She is a development communication specialist in program planning and research and development in population and health, sanitation and hygiene education, basic education, HIV/AIDS and adolescent reproductive health, and gender equity in South Asia and Africa. She has wide experience in managing entertainment-education projects in multicultural environments and was in charge of UNICEF's Sara Communication Initiative in Nairobi. Currently she is a communication officer with UNICEF, Kathmandu, and heads the Meena Communication Initiative.

Arvind Singhal is Presidential Research Scholar and professor in the School of Communication Studies, Ohio University, where he teaches and conducts research in the diffusion of innovations, mobilization for change, design and implementation of strategic communication campaigns, and entertainment-education communication strategy. He has authored or edited five books, including *Combating AIDS: Communication Strategies in Action*. He has researched and taught in more than forty countries.

D. Dow Tang is an undergraduate student at Yale University, majoring in political science. He has done voluntary work with Earthwatch and has sponsored the poultry projects of the Zienzele Foundation in Zimbabwe.

Shereen Usdin, a communication specialist in health and development, holds an M.D. from the University of the Witwatersrand Medical School and an M.P.H. from Harvard University. She cofounded the Soul City Institute for Health and Development Communication, where she is a senior manager, heading the *Soul City* series as well as the advocacy department. She has been a health and human rights activist for two decades and consults internationally in the health communications. She also sits on the board of many NGOs involved in human rights, gender-based violence, and health.

Kwardua Vanderpuye, who holds an M.P.H. from Columbia University, is a public health programs specialist with expertise in participatory training methodologies. She runs a consulting practice, CatalySis Consulting, in New York City and is a doctoral candidate in nonprofit management at Case Western Reserve University.

Kiragu Wambuii is a Ph.D. candidate and doctoral associate in political science at Western Michigan University. Born and raised on the scenic slopes of Mt. Kenya, his area of concentration is comparative politics, and his research interests lie in the sociopolitical sphere of development issues.

Index of Names

Index of Subjects

Note: Page numbers in italics refer to illustrations.